Nurse's Pocket Guide

Stewart Clark

Nursing Interaction

In 1958, Ida Jean Orlando began the nursing system that actually directs nursing care today. Characterized as an efficient way to deal with care utilizing the major standards of decisive reasoning, client-focused ways to deal with treatment, objective situated errands, proof based practice (EDP) suggestions, and nursing instinct. Comprehensive and logical hypothesizes are coordinated to give the premise to empathetic, quality-based care.

Capability

The nursing system capabilities as a precise manual for client-focused care with 5 consecutive advances. These are appraisal, determination, arranging, execution, and assessment. The first step, assessment, requires critical thinking skills and data collection; emotional and objective. Abstract information includes verbal proclamations from the patient or guardian. Objective information is quantifiable, unmistakable information like essential signs, admission and result, and level and weight. Data may be obtained directly from the patient or from primary caregivers, who may or may not be family members. Companions can assume a part in information assortment. Electronic wellbeing records might populate information and aid appraisal. Decisive reasoning abilities are vital for appraisal, subsequently the requirement for idea based educational plan changes.

The North American Nursing Determination Affiliation (NANDA) gives nurture a forward-thinking rundown of nursing analyze. According to NANDA, a nursing diagnosis is a clinical judgment regarding the patient, family, or community's responses to actual or potential health issues.

A nursing conclusion incorporates Maslow's Pecking order of Necessities and assists with focusing on and plan care in light of patient-focused results. In 1943, Abraham Maslow fostered a pecking order in view of essential thing needs natural to all people. Essential physiological requirements/objectives should be met before higher necessities/objectives can be accomplished like confidence and self-realization. Physiological and security needs give the premise to the execution of nursing care and nursing intercessions. Subsequently, they are at the foundation of Maslow's pyramid, establishing the groundwork for physical and profound health.

Fundamental Physiological Necessities: Nourishment (water and food), disposal (Toileting), aviation route (attractions)- breathing (oxygen)- dissemination (beat, heart screen, circulatory strain) (ABCs), rest, sex, asylum, and exercise.

Wellbeing and Security: Injury counteraction (side rails, call lights, hand cleanliness, seclusion, self-destruction safeguards, fall precautionary measures, vehicle seats, caps, safety belts), cultivating an environment of trust and security (remedial relationship), patient instruction (modifiable gamble factors for stroke, coronary illness).

Love and Having a place: Encourage steady connections, strategies to keep away from social detachment (harassing), utilize undivided attention procedures, restorative correspondence, and sexual closeness.

Self-Esteem: Acknowledgment locally, labor force, individual accomplishment, feeling of control or strengthening, tolerating one's actual appearance or body habitus.

Self-Actualization: Engaging climate, profound development, capacity to perceive the perspective of others, it one's greatest potential to reach.

Arranging

The arranging stage is where objectives and results are planned that straightforwardly influence patient consideration in light of EDP rules. The achievement of these patient-specific goals contributes to a positive outcome. In this stage of goal-setting, nursing care plans are essential. Care plans give a course of bearing to customized care custom-made to a singular's novel necessities. The development of a care plan is influenced in part by the patient's overall condition and other conditions. Care plans improve correspondence, documentation, repayment, and coherence of care across the medical services continuum.

The Following Ought To Be Objectives:

Execution

Execution is the step that includes activity or doing and the real completing of nursing mediations illustrated in the arrangement of care. This stage requires nursing mediations, for example, applying a cardiovascular screen or oxygen, immediate or circuitous consideration, prescription organization, standard treatment conventions, and EDP guidelines.

Assessment

This last step of the nursing system is crucial to a positive patient result. A healthcare provider must reevaluate or evaluate every time they intervene or provide care to ensure that the desired outcome has been achieved. Reassessment may often be required relying on by and large understanding condition. The arrangement of care might be adjusted in view of new appraisal information.

Issues of Concern

As per a recent report led in Mekelle Zone emergency clinics, medical caretakers come up short on information to execute the nursing system into training and factors, for example, nurture patient proportions restrain them from doing as such. A lot of study members needed adequate experience to apply the nursing system to standard practice. The concentrate likewise presumed that a deficiency of accessible assets, combined with expanded responsibilities because of high persistent medical caretaker proportions, added to the absence of the nursing system execution in the conveyance of patient care.

Clinical Importance

The use of the nursing system to direct mind is clinically critical proceeding in this unique, complex universe of patient consideration. Maturing populaces convey with them a large number of medical issues and intrinsic dangers of botched chances to recognize a life changing condition.

Salmond and Echevarria looked at how healthcare is changing and how nurses' traditional roles are changing to accommodate this new healthcare environment. Medical attendants are in a situation to advance change and effect patient conveyance care models in the future.

Different Issues

Decisive reasoning abilities will assume an essential part as we foster plans of care for these patient populaces with numerous comorbidities and embrace this difficult medical services field. Hence, the pattern towards idea based educational plan changes will help us in the route of these strange waters.

Idea Based Educational plan

Noble further investigates this requirement for an idea based educational plan rather than the conventional instructive model and the difficulties confronted with its execution. An immediate effect on quality patient consideration and positive results. Nursing practice and instructive conditions structure a bond with clinical information and skill, and that bond works with the progress into the ongoing labor force as a basic cooperative person and pioneer in this new rush of medical services.

Learning ought to be the concentration and the mix into current practice. Learning is a powerful cycle, moved by a power that should exist together inside a similar learning milieu among teacher and understudy, preceptor and beginner, guide, and student.

Later on, medical caretakers should have the option to issue tackle in a large number of circumstances and conditions to meet these new difficulties: testing attendant patient proportions, multi-layered ways to deal with prioritization of care, less assets, route of the electronic wellbeing record as well as usefulness inside the group dynamic and authority style.

A nursing diagnosis is a clinical judgment about how a person responds to health conditions or life processes, or how vulnerable they are to that response, by themselves, their family, group, or community. A nursing finding gives the premise to choosing nursing intercessions to accomplish results for which the medical caretaker has responsibility. Based on the information gathered during the nursing assessment, nursing diagnoses enable the nurse to create a care plan.

The term nursing analysis is related with various ideas. It could be a reference to the distinct second stage of the nursing process, diagnosis (the "D" in "ADPIE"). Likewise, nursing conclusion applies to the mark when medical caretakers dole out importance to gathered information suitably named a nursing determination. For instance, during the appraisal, the medical caretaker might perceive that the client feels restless, unfortunate, and finds it challenging to rest. Those issues are marked with nursing analyze: individually, Tension, Dread, and Upset Rest Example. In this specific situation, a nursing finding depends on the patient's reaction to the ailment. Because these are matters that hold a distinct and precise action associated with what nurses have the autonomy to take action about with a specific disease or condition, it is referred to as a "nursing diagnosis." Anything that elicits a mental, emotional, or spiritual response is included in this. Subsequently, a nursing determination is centered around care.

Then again, a clinical conclusion is made by the doctor or high level medical care specialist that manages the illness, ailment, or neurotic state just a professional can treat.

In addition, the doctor will, through experience and expertise, identify the specific and precise clinical entity that could be the illness's cause and prescribe the appropriate medication to treat it. Instances of clinical judgments are Diabetes Mellitus, Tuberculosis, Removal, Hepatitis, and Constant Kidney Illness. The clinical determination typically doesn't change. Medical caretakers should follow the doctor's requests and complete recommended therapies and treatments. Nurses can deal with collaborative issues by employing both self-prescribed and physician-prescribed interventions. These are issues or conditions that require both clinical and nursing intercessions, with the nursing angle zeroed in on observing the client's condition and forestalling the advancement of the possible complexity.

As made sense of above, presently recognizing a nursing determination from a clinical diagnosis is more straightforward. Nursing finding is coordinated towards the patient and their physiological and mental reaction. Then again, a clinical finding is specific to the infection or ailment. Its middle is on the sickness.

Nursing Cycle

The five phases of the nursing system are appraisal, diagnosing, arranging, execution, and assessment. All means in the nursing system require decisive reasoning by the medical caretaker. The nurse promotes awareness of the defining characteristics and behaviors of the diagnoses, related factors to the selected nursing diagnoses, and the interventions that are suitable for treating the diagnoses in addition to understanding the nursing diagnoses and their definitions.

Kinds of Nursing Analyses

The four kinds of nursing analysis are Real (Issue Centered), Hazard, Wellbeing Advancement, and Condition. The four types of nursing diagnoses are as follows:

Issue Centered Nursing Analysis

An issue centered finding (otherwise called real conclusion) is a client issue present at the hour of the nursing evaluation. These determinations depend on the presence of related signs and side effects. Genuine nursing analysis ought not be seen as more significant than risk analyze. There are many occasions where a gamble determination can be the finding with the most noteworthy need for a patient.

Issue centered nursing analyze have three parts:

1. Nursing determination
2. Related variables, and
3. Characterizing qualities. Instances of genuine nursing analyze are:

Acute pain related to decreased myocardial flow as evidenced by grimacing, expression of pain, and guarding behavior Anxiety related to stress as demonstrated by increased tension, apprehension, and expression of concern regarding upcoming surgery

Risk Nursing Diagnosis

Risk nursing diagnosis is the second type of nursing diagnosis. These are clinical decisions that an issue doesn't exist, yet the presence of hazard factors shows that an issue is probably going to foster except if medical caretakers mediate. A gamble determination depends on the patient's ongoing wellbeing status, past wellbeing history, and other gamble factors that might improve the patient's probability of encountering a medical condition. Because they enable the nurse to take measures to either prevent or reduce the risk, these are an essential part of nursing care. They also aid in the early detection of potential issues.

For risk diagnoses, there are no etiological (related) factors. The individual (or gathering) is more vulnerable to fostering the issue than others in the equivalent or a comparative circumstance due to gamble with factors. For instance, if an elderly client has diabetes and vertigo and has trouble walking but refuses to ask for help while ambulating, they may be correctly diagnosed as being at risk of injury or falling.

Risk for Injury and Disease

Wellbeing Advancement Determination

Wellbeing advancement determination (otherwise called health finding) is a clinical judgment about inspiration and want to increment prosperity. An assertion recognizes the patient's preparation for taking part in exercises that advance wellbeing and prosperity. For instance, in the event that a first-time mother tells interest on the best way to appropriately breastfeed her child, a medical caretaker make a wellbeing advancement conclusion of "Status for Upgraded Breastfeeding." This nursing analysis will be then used to direct nursing mediations pointed toward supporting the patient in finding out about appropriate breastfeeding.

Additionally, the individual, family, or community's transition from a particular level of wellness to a higher level of wellness is the focus of health promotion diagnosis. Parts of a wellbeing advancement conclusion by and large incorporate just the indicative mark or a one-section proclamation. Instances of wellbeing advancement finding:

Condition Conclusion

A condition conclusion is a clinical judgment concerning a group of issue or chance nursing analyze that are anticipated to introduce due to a specific circumstance or occasion. They, as well, are composed as a one-section explanation requiring just the demonstrative mark. Instances of a condition nursing finding are:

Constant Torment Disorder

Conceivable Nursing Conclusion

A potential nursing determination isn't a sort of conclusion as are real, risk, wellbeing advancement, and condition. Statements describing a suspected problem for which additional data are required to either confirm or rule out the suspected problem are known as possible nursing diagnoses. It furnishes the medical caretaker with the capacity to speak with different medical attendants that a conclusion might be available however extra information assortment is demonstrated to preclude or affirm the determination.

Issue and Definition

The issue explanation, or the analytic mark, portrays the client's medical condition or reaction to which nursing treatment is given succinctly. A symptomatic name generally has two sections: focus and qualifier of the diagnosis. Words that have been added to some diagnostic labels to give the statement more meaning, limit, or specify it are referred to as qualifiers (also known as modifiers). One-word nursing diagnoses, such as anxiety, constipation, diarrhea, and nausea, are exempt from this rule. where the single term serves as both their qualifier and focus.

Sustenance

Sustenance, the osmosis by living creatures of food materials that empower them to develop, keep up with themselves, and duplicate. Food serves different capabilities in most living organic entities. It provides, for instance, materials that are metabolized in order to supply the energy required for the absorption and translocation of nutrients, the synthesis of cell materials, movement and locomotion, the elimination of waste products, and all other organismal activities. All of the structural and catalytic components of a living cell can be assembled from the materials provided by food as well. Living creatures contrast in the specific substances that they expect as food, in how they combine food substances or acquire them from the general climate, and in the capabilities that these substances complete in their cells. Nevertheless, the nutritional processes of all living things and the kinds of nutrients that are necessary for life can be identified in general patterns. These examples are the subject of this article. For a full conversation of the dietary prerequisites of people specifically, see the article sustenance, human.

Wholesome Examples in the Living Scene

Living organic entities can be classified by the manner by which the elements of food are done in their bodies. Subsequently, creatures, for example, green plants and a few microbes that need just inorganic mixtures for development can be called autotrophic organic entities; what's more, organic entities, including all creatures, parasites, and most microbes, that require both inorganic and natural mixtures for development are called heterotrophic. Different characterizations have been utilized to incorporate different other healthful examples. In one plan, creatures are characterized by the energy source they use. Phototrophic, or photosynthetic, organic entities trap light energy and convert it to substance energy, though chemoautotrophic, or chemosynthetic, organic entities use inorganic or natural mixtures to supply their energy prerequisites. Assuming the electron-giver materials used to shape decreased coenzymes comprise of inorganic mixtures, the life form is supposed to be lithotrophic; if natural, the creature is organotrophic.

Mixes of these examples may likewise be utilized to depict life forms. Higher plants, for instance, are photolithotrophic; i.e., they use light energy, with the inorganic compound water filling in as a definitive electron contributor. Certain photosynthetic microbes that can't use water as the electron giver and require natural mixtures for this inspiration are called photoorganotrophs. Creatures, as indicated by this order, are chemoorganotrophs; i.e., they use substance mixtures to supply energy and natural mixtures as electron benefactors.

All organisms derive an immediate source of energy from their external energy source, the chemical compound adenosine triphosphate (ATP), despite the numerous variations in the nature of the external energy source utilized by various organisms. This energy-rich compound is normal to all cells. Through the breaking of its high-energy phosphate bonds and consequently by its transformation to a less energy-rich compound, adenosine diphosphate (ADP), ATP gives the energy to the substance and mechanical work expected by a life form. Either joules or calories can be used to measure an organism's energy needs.

Sustenance in Plants

Plants, in contrast to creatures, don't need to acquire natural materials for their sustenance, albeit these structure the majority of their tissues. By catching sun powered energy in photosynthetic frameworks, they can combine supplements from carbon dioxide (CO_2) and water. But plants do need inorganic salts, which they get from the soil around their roots; these incorporate the components phosphorus (as phosphate), chlorine (as the chloride particle), potassium, sulfur, calcium, magnesium, iron, manganese, boron, copper, and zinc. Plants additionally require nitrogen, as nitrate (NO_3^-) or ammonium (NH_4^+) particles. They will, also, take up inorganic mixtures that they personally don't require, for example, iodides and cobalt and selenium salts.

The supplements found in soil bring about part from the continuous breakdown of the rough material on Earth's surface because of downpour and, in certain areas, freezing. Basically made out of alumina and silica, shakes likewise contain more modest measures of the multitude of mineral components required by plants. One more wellspring of soil supplements is the disintegration of dead plants and creatures and their side-effects. Albeit a spadeful of soil might appear to be idle to the eye — aside from an incidental night crawler — it contains a great many microorganisms, the net impact of which is to separate natural materials, delivering less difficult mineral salts. Moreover, two gatherings of microbes fix air nitrogen — that is, they can integrate this somewhat latent component into nitrate particles. Microbes of the class Azobacter live unreservedly in soil, while those of the variety Rhizobium live protected in the underlying foundations of leguminous plants like peas and beans. Cyanobacteria (blue green growth) additionally can fix nitrogen and are significant for developing rice in the overflowed paddy fields of Southeast Asia.

Human intervention in the form of fertilizers is crucial in areas of intensive farming where crops are harvested at least once a year and no animals roam the fields. Animal manure, or muck, is a traditional fertilizer made from cattle bedding straw that has been soaked in excrement and allowed to ferment for some time. Farmers have also used artificial fertilizers since the 1800s, beginning with naturally occurring chemical mixtures like chalk (which provides calcium), rock phosphates, and natural guano. Business guano comprises of the amassed stores of bird droppings and is esteemed for its high grouping of nitrates. Present day synthetic manures incorporate at least one of three significant components: nitrogen, potassium, and phosphorus. Most nitrogenous manures are delivered by a strategy in which nitrogen and hydrogen are consolidated at extremely high constrains within the sight of impetuses to shape smelling salts (NH3). This can then be infused into the dirt as a gas that is immediately retained or, all the more regularly, changed over into strong items, for example, ammonium salts, urea, and nitrates, which can be utilized as fixings in blended composts.

Nourishment in Microscopic Organisms

These little creatures, famously considered exclusively as wellsprings of disease, are of imperative significance in the general life patterns of plants and creatures. As with larger organisms, they frequently have to digest their food, and their cell walls prevent the passage of large compounds. Sugars will diffuse through the bacterial wall into larger molecules as a result of the concentration gradient continuing to encourage inward diffusion if the bacteria are in a sugar-containing liquid. In any case, to use bigger particles, for example, starches and protein, microscopic organisms need to discharge stomach related compounds (i.e., impetuses) into the encompassing liquid. This is clearly a costly function for a single organism because a lot of the digested products and enzymes that are secreted may drift away from the bacterial cell rather than toward it. Be that as it may, for a bunch of thousands or millions of microorganisms acting similarly, the cycle is more affordable.

Microorganisms change enormously in their dietary prerequisites. Some, similar to plants, require a wellspring of energy like sugars and just inorganic supplements. Some are high-impact, implying that they require oxygen to catch energy — for instance, by oxidation of sugars to carbon dioxide and water. Others are anaerobic, which means they are actually poisoned by oxygen, and they need an energy source like sugar, which they can ferment into lactic acid or ethanol and carbon dioxide to get enough energy to meet their needs.

Evidently as a transformation to numerous ages of living in a supplement rich medium, a microorganisms have lost the capacity to blend numerous fundamental mixtures. For instance, a considerable lot of the Lactobacilli, normally tracked down in unsterilized milk, require basically every one of the water-dissolvable nutrients and amino acids required by creatures. Along these lines, they have been utilized as helpful models for measuring the worth of food varieties as wellsprings of specific supplements.

Sustenance in Creatures

Basic perception uncovers that the collective of animals is subject to plants for food. Indeed, even meat-eating, or rapacious, creatures, for example, the lion feed on touching creatures and accordingly are in a roundabout way subject to the plant realm for their endurance.

Herbivores

Plant cell walls are developed predominantly of cellulose, a material that the stomach related compounds of higher creatures can't process or disturb. Along these lines, even the nutritious items in plant cells are not completely accessible for processing. As a developmental reaction to this issue, many leaf eaters, or herbivores, have fostered a pocket at the front finish of the stomach, called the rumen, that gives a space to the bacterial maturation of ingested leaves. In ruminant species like cows and sheep, aged material, called cud, is disgorged from the rumen so the creature can bite it into considerably more modest pieces and spread the ruminal liquid all through the mass of ingesta. Microorganisms found in the ruminal liquid mature cellulose to acidic corrosive and other short-chain unsaturated fats, which can then be consumed and used as energy sources. Protein inside the cells of the leaves is additionally delivered and debased; In the true stomach and small intestine, some of it is resynthesized into microbial protein for digestion. One more activity of ruminal microscopic organisms is the amalgamation of a few water-dissolvable nutrients so that, under most circumstances, the host creature no longer expects them to be provided in its food.

Since conditions in the rumen are anaerobic, one more impact of ruminal maturation is that the greasy material in the food becomes hydrogenated. In many organisms' metabolic reactions, hydrogen atoms are removed. If the hydrogen that is left over can't be combined with oxygen to make water, it can be added to unsaturated fatty acids. The outcome is more immersed unsaturated fats, which, after retention, structure stores of more earnestly fat. Consequently, hamburger fat (suet) is typically more diligently at room temperature than is pork or chicken fat. The addition of short-chain fatty acids to the glycerol esters keeps butterfat somewhat soft at room temperature, keeping it similarly relatively saturated. This absence of the fundamental polyunsaturated unsaturated fats in ruminant fats can make them less alluring as human food.

Different herbivores take advantage of verdant food varieties through hindgut aging. In creature species for the most part, the fundamental breakdown of food sources by chemicals and assimilation into the circulatory system happens in the small digestive tract. When there is a limited supply of water, the large intestine's primary function is to absorb the majority of the remaining water to reduce losses. In the "hindgut fermenters," undigested food buildups go through bacterial maturation in the cecum, a side pocket at the distal finish of the small digestive tract, prior to moving into the internal organ. The cecum's short-chain fatty acids are absorbed and utilized in the large intestine. Horses, zebras, elephants, rhinoceroses, koalas, and rabbits are among the animals in this category.

Hindgut fermenters are to some degree less productive than are ruminants at processing exceptionally high-fiber food varieties. However, the cecum only ferments indigestible residues, preventing hindgut fermenters from experiencing the inevitable loss of energy that occurs when dietary carbohydrates ferment in the rumen. Likewise, the more modest main part of the cecum permits these creatures to be more athletic and better ready to get away from their flesh eater hunters.

Carnivores

Carnivores fundamentally structure just a little part of the set of all animals, in light of the fact that every creature should eat a large number of different creatures of identical size to keep up with itself over a long period. Carnivores not only have the teeth and claws they need to kill and tear their prey apart, but they also have digestive enzymes that can break down muscle protein into amino acids that can then diffuse through the small intestine's walls.

Hence, carnivores have no requirement for any exceptional advancement of the stomach that takes into consideration aging. Carnivores are likewise ready to use creature fat. In the event that their prey is little, they can bite and swallow bones, which act as a wellspring of calcium. A few carnivores, especially felines (family Felidae), are commit carnivores, meaning they can't get every one of the supplements that they need from the plant realm and microorganisms. Specifically, commit carnivores miss the mark on compound expected to part carotene, got from plants, into vitamin A. All things considered, these creatures get vitamin A from the liver of their prey. Commit carnivores are likewise unfit to blend some fundamental extremely lengthy chain, exceptionally unsaturated fats that different creatures can make from more limited unsaturated fats tracked down in plants.

Omnivores

Omnivores are different species whose teeth and stomach related frameworks appear to be intended to eat a somewhat thought diet, since they have no enormous sac or chamber for the maturation of sinewy material. They can chew and digest meat, but they don't absolutely need it unless they can't get it from other sources of vitamin B12 (cobalamin). People are in this classification, as are canines, rodents, and most monkeys. In their small cecum and large intestine, all omnivores have active bacterial flora. At this point, they are able to absorb short-chain fatty acids but not vitamins. A few animal categories get fundamental nutrients by coprophagy, the eating of an extent of their waste pellets that contain nutrients combined by microorganisms. Chickens, as well, are omnivores. They must swallow food without chewing it; however, the food travels to the gizzard, an organ where seeds and other foods are ground into a slurry frequently with the assistance of swallowed stones.

Supplements

A few forerunners (i.e., the substances from which different substances are framed) of cell materials can be combined by the cell from different materials, while others should be provided in food varieties. The latter category includes all of the inorganic materials necessary for growth as well as a variety of organic compounds whose numbers can range from one to thirty or more, depending on the organism. Even though organisms are capable of synthesizing nonessential nutrients, these nutrients are frequently utilized directly when they are present in food, saving the organism the energy required to synthesize them.

Inorganic supplements

Various inorganic components (minerals) are fundamental for the development of living things. Boron, for instance, has been shown to be expected for the development of numerous — maybe all — higher plants yet has not been embroiled as a fundamental component in the nourishment of either microorganisms or creatures. Follow measures of fluorine (as fluoride) are unquestionably advantageous, and maybe fundamental, for appropriate tooth development in higher creatures. In a similar vein, animals need iodine (as iodide) to make thyroxine, an important regulatory hormone's active component. Silicon, also known as silicate, is required for normal growth in diatomaceous protozoans and other similar organisms because it is a prominent component of their outer skeletons. In higher creatures the prerequisite for silicon is a lot more modest. A more subtle illustration of a particular mineral necessity is given by calcium, which is expected by higher creatures in similarly enormous sums since it is a significant part of bone and eggshells (in birds); for different living beings, calcium is a fundamental supplement yet just as a minor component. Mineral components in wide assortment are available in follow sums in practically all staples. It can't be accepted that the unimportant mineral components assume no valuable part in digestion.

Significant hostile connections between specific mineral supplements likewise are known. An enormous overabundance of rubidium, for instance, impedes the use of potassium in a few lactic-corrosive microbes; zinc can slow down manganese use in a similar living being. In creature nourishment, over the top molybdenum or zinc (the two of which are fundamental minerals) disrupts the use of copper, another fundamental mineral, and, in higher plants, exorbitant zinc can prompt a problem that is known as iron chlorosis. Therefore, not only must sufficient amounts of the essential mineral elements be provided, but they must also be used in the appropriate ratios to one another in order to make appropriate nutrient growth media for plants, microorganisms, and animals.

Organic nutrients Organic nutrients are the building blocks of various cell parts that some organisms can't make and must get from other sources. These mixtures incorporate carbs, protein, and lipids. Vitamins are another organic nutrient that is required in small quantities due to either their catalytic or regulatory functions in metabolism.

Sugars

Quantitatively, the most significant of supplements are the sugars orchestrated by plants, since they give the greater part of the energy used by the collective of animals. Mature organic product is wealthy in sugars that draw in birds and other little creatures. The seed coats in the organic product endure their quick entry through the stomach of these creatures, who accordingly disperse broadly the still suitable seeds of the plant. Sucrose, specifically, additionally amasses in the stems of sugarcane and in the underlying foundations of sugar beet, filling in as an energy save for each plant; both are utilized for the modern creation of table sugar.

Dietary sugars incorporate monosaccharides, which contain one sugar (glucose) unit, and disaccharides, which are comprised of two sugar units connected together. To be used by a creature, all mind boggling carbs should be separated into basic sugars, which, by and large, are quickly processed and ingested. For instance, even the uninhibitedly dissolvable disaccharide sucrose should initially be hydrolyzed to glucose and fructose by a particular catalyst, sucrase. Infant piglets don't emit this compound and hence can't utilize sucrose. Alternately, the disaccharide lactose is quickly hydrolyzed by infant creatures, however most species — even a few people — quit emitting the chemical lactase in the wake of weaning. This is justifiable since lactose happens normally just in milk, which a creature as a rule won't experience again after its nursing period.

The significant stockpiling sugar in plant seeds, starch is a polysaccharide, framed from the buildup of a few glucose units, fundamentally through linkages that are quickly broken somewhere near stomach related proteins in microorganisms as well as in higher creatures. Nonetheless, unique plant starches fluctuate in the cross-linkages between these fundamental chains, and this variety can bring about additional conservative atoms that are impervious to assimilation. One of the significant impacts of cooking is that starch granules enlarge with consumed water and become all the more effectively edible. Surprisingly, even members of the cat family, who do not consume starch in their natural diet as carnivores, can make good use of it when ground finely. Business dry feline food sources might contain 20% or more starch.

Plant cell walls are built chiefly from cellulose. Similar to starch, cellulose is made from condensed glucose units. However, a different kind of linkage allows the chains to lie flat, and vertebrates do not have enzymes that can digest these linkages. However, herbivorous species have gastrointestinal systems that enable the bacterial fermentation of cellulose in either the rumen (foregut) or the hindgut (rumen), allowing the animals to benefit from cellulose metabolites, particularly short-chain fatty acids. Different polysaccharides in plant cell walls incorporate gelatins and hemicelluloses, which give a combination of sugars, like xylose and arabinose, upon hydrolysis. These sugars additionally are aged by microbes however are not separated and processed by creature catalysts. Inflexible plant structures contain lignin, a phenolic polymer that is impenetrable to processing by the two creatures and microbes. Thought about together, these materials make up what is called dietary fiber.

Lipids (Fats and Oils)

One more structure in which a few plants store energy in their seeds is fat, generally called oil in its fluid structure. In creatures, fats structure the main huge scope energy store. Compared to carbohydrates, fats provide a more concentrated source of energy. oxidation yields about nine and four kilocalories of energy for each gram, individually.

Three fatty acids attached to a glycerol backbone make up a fat, which is a hydrocarbon chain with a carboxylic acid group at one end. The actual properties of fats rely upon the unsaturated fats that they contain. All fats are fluid when present in living tissues. The fats of warm-blooded creatures can, obviously, have a higher edge of freezing over than that of unfeeling creatures like fish. Plants that endure ices should have an especially low edge of freezing over. In most cases, organisms store fat with little or no excess liquid in it; that is, it has an edge of freezing over close to the greatest steady with the organic entity's feasibility.

Unsaturated fats vary from each other in two ways: length of the chain and saturation The majority of fatty acids have 16 or 18 carbons in their chain length, which ranges from 4 to 22. The generally low edge of freezing over of a cow's butterfat results from its substance of the 4-carbon short-chain unsaturated fat butyric corrosive; The acids and the fat that contains them have a lower freezing point the longer the saturated chains are. Notwithstanding, a more prominent impact of liquidity comes from the presentation of unsaturated (twofold) securities in the chains. More than one twofold bond (polyunsaturation) makes it more hard for fats to stay strong at room temperature.

Fatty acids taken in by animals are typically stored or immediately oxidized for energy. Specific unsaturated fats are required for the development of phospholipids, which structure a fundamental piece of cell layers and nerve filaments, and for the combination of specific chemicals. Creatures can combine their own fat from an overabundance of retained sugars, yet they are restricted in their capacity to orchestrate fundamental polyunsaturated unsaturated fats, for example, linoleic corrosive and linolenic corrosive. In this manner, unsaturated fats are not only an elective energy source — they are a fundamental dietary fixing. Linoleic acid can be found in a small amount in the majority of vegetable oils, which are also good sources of linoleic acid. Felines have lost one of the chief chemicals utilized by different creatures to change over linoleic corrosive to arachidonic corrosive, which is required for the blend of prostaglandins and different chemicals. Since arachidonic corrosive isn't found in plants, felines are commit carnivores, really intending that under normal circumstances they should eat creature tissue to make due and recreate.

Proteins

The vitally natural material in the functioning tissue of the two plants and creatures is protein, huge atoms containing chains of dense units of around 20 different amino acids. Before entering the bloodstream, animal protein food is digested into free amino acids. As long as they have access to nitrate or other simple nitrogenous compounds and sulfur, which is required for the synthesis of cysteine and methionine, plants are able to produce their own amino acids, which are necessary for the production of proteins. Ammonium ions and carbohydrate metabolites can also be used by animals to make some amino acids; be that as it may, others can't be incorporated and are thusly dietary basics. Two amino acids, cysteine and tyrosine, can be orchestrated simply by digestion of the fundamental amino acids methionine and phenylalanine, separately. Microscopic organisms living in the rumen of ruminant creatures can orchestrate every one of the amino acids usually present in protein, and the genuine stomach of the ruminant will keep on getting microbial protein of sensibly great quality for assimilation.

Protein helps animals grow. This necessity is generally relative to the development rate and is reflected in the protein content of the milk discharged during the nursing time frame. For instance, a piglet copies its introduction to the world load in 18 days, and sow's milk has protein at a level providing 25% of the all out energy. Conversely, people require roughly 180 days to twofold their introduction to the world weight, and bosom milk contains protein at a level identical to something like 8% of the all out energy. Youthful creatures took care of trial eats less totally inadequate with regards to one fundamental amino corrosive all display a quick discontinuance of development.

Grown-ups, as well, require protein in genuinely huge sums, more than would be expected to supplant the limited quantity of protein lost by the body through pee, defecation, and shed hair and skin. The facts really confirm that creature tissues are consistently "turning over" their proteins — i.e., hydrolyzing and once again integrating them — yet this doesn't make sense of the extra protein prerequisite, since the amino acids delivered are accessible for reuse. It shows up, in any case, that the compounds accessible to utilize abundance amino acids don't inactivate totally when the body is shy of protein however rather stay at an "standing by" rate. Ordinarily, this isn't an inconvenience, since the eating regimens of grown-up creatures, including people, contain more protein than is expected to adjust the standing by misfortunes. It likewise creates the impression that, over development, the sitting rates have become generally acclimated to the typical protein admission. Hence, grown-up rodents living on a scope of food varieties — some very low in protein — need something like 5% of their energy as protein. Conversely, felines, whose tribal savage eating regimen was a lot higher in protein, need nearly 20% in their eating regimen to adjust negligible misfortunes.

Nutrients

Nutrients might be characterized as natural substances that assume an expected reactant part inside the cell (typically as parts of coenzymes or different gatherings related with proteins) and should be gotten in limited quantities through the eating regimen. Nutrient necessities are explicit for every living being, and their inadequacy might cause sickness. Young animals with vitamin deficiencies typically experience stunted growth, a variety of symptoms whose nature is dependent on the vitamin, and ultimately death.

Albeit a nutrient is normally characterized as a natural synthetic which a creature or human should get from the eating routine in tiny sums, this isn't completely evident. Except for cats and probably other carnivores, which must obtain the preformed vitamin by consuming the tissues of other animals under natural conditions, most animals are able to split a molecule of carotene into two molecules of vitamin A. Although the pigment carotene is universally present in green plants, vitamin A does not exist in the plant kingdom. The majority of animals, with the exception of cats, are able to synthesize niacin from the amino acid tryptophan if tryptophan is present in excess of its use for protein synthesis.

Vitamin D is certainly not a genuine nutrient: most species don't require it in their eating routine, since they get a sufficient stock through the openness of skin to daylight, which switches a sterol present in dermal tissue over completely to vitamin D. The nutrient is hence processed to frame a chemical that demonstrations to control the ingestion and use of calcium and phosphate. Creatures, for example, rodents, which typically have little openness to daylight and quest for food generally around evening time, seem to have advanced to be autonomous of vitamin D inasmuch as their admissions of calcium and phosphate are even.

L-ascorbic acid (ascorbic corrosive) is a fundamental compound in the tissues, everything being equal, however most can make it for themselves, so that for them it's anything but a nutrient. Humans, guinea pigs, and fruit-eating bats are among the species that cannot synthesize vitamin C. It is likely that their ancestors lost this ability when their diet was high in ascorbic acid.

Vitamin requirements vary greatly between bacteria. Many are completely autonomous of outside sources, however at the other outrageous a portion of the kinds of microorganisms tracked down in milk (i.e., Lactobacillus) have lost the capacity to orchestrate the B nutrients that they need. This property has made them helpful for examining concentrates of food varieties for their vitamin B content. To be sure, numerous nutrients of this gathering were first found as development factors for microbes prior to being tried with creatures and people. The blended bacterial vegetation in the guts of creatures are, on balance, synthesizers of the B nutrients. Subsequently, ruminant creatures don't need to get them from an outside source. Then again, the capacity of hindgut fermenters to ingest nutrients from their internal organ is dubious. Rodents and bunnies, whose dietary necessities have been concentrated seriously, have both been found to take part in coprophagy, the eating of waste pellets that are nutrient rich because of bacterial aging in the hindgut.

For one B nutrient — cobalamin, or vitamin B12 — bacterial maturation is the main source, however it very well may be gotten in a roundabout way from the tissues or milk of creatures that have gotten it themselves from microorganisms. The speculation that "the set of all animals lives on the plant realm" is hence not every bit of relevant information, since creatures depend part of the way on microorganisms for this one micronutrient.

Interdependency of Nourishing Necessities

The impacts of one mineral supplement in diminishing or expanding the necessity for another have been referenced already. Comparative connections happen among natural supplements and start in light of multiple factors, the most widely recognized of which are examined momentarily underneath.

Since retention of supplements habitually happens via dynamic vehicle inside cell films, an overabundance of one supplement (A) may repress ingestion of a subsequent supplement (B), in the event that they share a similar retention pathway. The apparent requirement for nutrient B rises in such instances; B, nonetheless, can in some cases be provided in an other structure that can enter the cell by an alternate course. Numerous instances of amino corrosive enmity, where restraint of development by one amino corrosive is checked by one more amino corrosive, are best made sense of by this component. For instance, under certain circumstances Lactobacillus casei requires both D-and L-alanine, which contrast from one another main in the place of the amino, or NH2, bunch in the particle, and the two types of this amino corrosive offer a similar retention pathway. Overabundance D-alanine hinders development of this species, yet the restraint can be eased either by providing extra L-alanine or, all the more really, by providing peptides of L-alanine. The peptides enter the cell by a pathway not quite the same as that of the two types of alanine and, after they are in the cell, can be separated to frame L-alanine. One possible explanation for the fact that peptides frequently outperform amino acids in promoting the growth of bacteria is the existence of relationships of this kind.

Competition within the cell for utilization sites is similar to competition for absorption sites, but it only takes place within the cell between nutrients that are structurally similar (like leucine and valine; serine and threonine).

Antecedent Item Connections

The necessity of rodents and people for the fundamental amino acids phenylalanine and methionine is significantly decreased if tyrosine, which is shaped from phenylalanine, or cysteine, which is framed from methionine, is added to the eating routine. These connections are made sense of by the way that tyrosine and cysteine are blended in creatures from phenylalanine and methionine, separately. At the point when the previous (item) amino acids are provided preformed, the last option (antecedent) amino acids are expected in more modest sums. A few occasions of the saving of one supplement by another on the grounds that they have comparable forerunner item connections have been distinguished in different creatures.

Changes in Metabolic Pathways inside the Cell

Rodents took care of diets containing a lot of fat require significantly less thiamin (vitamin B1) than do those took care of diets high in sugar. The use of sugar as an energy source (i.e., for ATP development) is known to include a significant thiamin-subordinate step, which is avoided when fat is utilized as an energy source, and it is accepted that the diminished necessity for thiamin results from the adjustment of metabolic pathways.

Syntrophism

Since the dietary prerequisites and metabolic exercises of creatures contrast, obviously at least two distinct organic entities developing relatedly may deliver different generally speaking changes in the climate.

An unpleasant model is given by a fair aquarium, in which oceanic plants use light and the side-effects of creatures — e.g., carbon dioxide, water, smelling salts — to combine cell materials and produce oxygen, which thus give the materials important to creature development. Such connections are normal among microorganisms; i.e., middle or finished results of digestion of one living being might give fundamental supplements to another. This phenomenon, which is known as syntrophism, can be seen in nature's mixed populations; Nutritional symbiosis, or mutualism, may occur when the relationship is so close to being mutual. A few instances of this peculiarity have been found among thiamin-requiring yeasts and organisms, sure of which (bunch A) combined the thiazole part of thiamin particle yet require the pyrimidine segment preformed; briefly bunch (bunch B), the relationship is switched. Because each organism synthesizes the growth factor required by its partner, both groups of organisms survive when grown together in a medium devoid of thiamin; neither one of the life forms develops alone under these equivalent circumstances. In this way, at least two sorts of microorganisms much of the time fill in circumstances in which only one animal groups wouldn't.

Such wholesome interrelationships might make sense of the way that the healthfully requesting lactic-corrosive microbes can coincide with the healthfully nondemanding coliform microscopic organisms in the digestive systems of creatures. It is realized that the bacterial verdure of the digestive system combine adequate measures of specific nutrients (e.g., vitamin K, folic corrosive) so identification of lack side effects in rodents requires unique measures, and the job of rumen microbes in ruminant creatures (e.g., cows, sheep) in delivering in any case unpalatable cellulose and different materials accessible to the host creature is notable. These couple of models demonstrate that syntrophic interrelationships are far reaching in nature and may contribute considerably to the nourishment of a wide assortment of animal varieties.

Dietary Advancement of Organic Entities

Little is had some significant awareness of the dietary advancement of living organic entities. All living cells contain nucleic acids, proteins, carbohydrates, and fats that are created through specific reaction sequences from a small number of smaller compounds. The majority of these smaller compounds are common to all living organisms and, according to current theories, existed on Earth long before life emerged. Since synthesizing cellular proteins from preformed amino acids requires less energy and less complex metabolic organization than synthesizing proteins from carbon dioxide or other precursors, it is assumed that the simplest early forms of life were heterotrophic organisms that selected organic nutrients from their surroundings. As the stock of these preformed substances was depleted, the creatures probably fostered the ability to blend these preformed substances from easier (forerunner) materials present in the climate; in certain organic entities, this blending limit in the long run advanced to the degree that carbon from carbon dioxide could be used to orchestrate natural mixtures.

Autotrophy, as it is now known, became possible at this point; autotrophy, as a matter of fact, may have developed because of the fatigue of the stockpile of preformed natural materials in the climate and the subsequent need of life forms to blend the actual necessities to make due. Implied in this hypothesis is the evident supposition that autotrophic cells contain the most mind boggling biosynthetic association found in living things and that heterotrophic cells are less complex in that specific biosynthetic pathways don't happen. After the development of photosynthesis, a continually sustainable wellspring of the natural mixtures important for heterotrophic cell development opened up. It became possible that those organic entities whose conditions gave a continually accessible stockpile of a given compound could lose, through changes in their hereditary material (transformations), the capacity to combine that compound regardless make due. Whole biosynthetic pathways might have been lost along these lines; Using preformed cell components would have saved energy and given mutant organisms a competitive advantage over the more complex parents from which they were derived, allowing them to stabilize the mutation within the cell type as long as they were in an environment that provided the necessary compound. A hypothesis that the prerequisites of current creatures for fundamental natural supplements emerged through the deficiency of engineered capacities present in more perplexing guardian organic entities was affirmed by the disclosure that falsely delivered freak posterity of microorganisms can be promptly gotten and may require the presence of at least one preformed natural mixtures that the parent microorganisms could combine.

Human Sustenance

Human sustenance, process by which substances in food are changed into body tissues and give energy to the full scope of physical and mental exercises that make up human existence.

In addition to physiology, biochemistry, and molecular biology, the study of human nutrition involves psychology and anthropology, which investigate how attitudes, beliefs, preferences, and cultural traditions influence food choices. As the world community acknowledges and responds to the suffering and death caused by malnutrition, human nutrition further touches on economics and political science. A definitive objective of dietary science is to advance ideal wellbeing and decrease the gamble of persistent illnesses, for example, cardiovascular sickness and malignant growth as well as to forestall exemplary wholesome inadequacy infections like kwashiorkor and pellagra.

The most important aspects of human nutrition are discussed in this article, including the balance and generation of energy, essential nutrients, and suggested dietary guidelines. For a full-length treatment of medical conditions made by disappointment in nourishment, see dietary illness. The use of food materials by all living things is depicted in nourishment, and explicit biochemical cycles are portrayed in digestion.

Usage of Food by the Body

Calories and kilocalories

The human body can be considered a motor that delivers the energy present in the food sources that it digests. This energy is used part of the way for the mechanical work performed by the muscles and in the secretory cycles and part of the way for the work important to keep up with the body's construction and capabilities. The presentation of work is related with the development of intensity; heat misfortune is controlled in order to keep internal heat level inside a limited reach. However, in contrast to other engines, the human body constantly decomposes (catabolizes) and builds up (anabolizes) its components. Food varieties supply supplements fundamental for the production of the new material and give energy expected to the synthetic responses included. Comprehend the idea of calorie, the utilization of dietary benefit on the food mark, and techniques to gauge them

Sugar, fat, and protein are, generally, compatible as wellsprings of energy. Normally, the energy given by food is estimated in kilocalories, or Calories. One kilocalorie is equivalent to 1,000 gram-calories (or little calories), a proportion of intensity energy. Nonetheless, in like manner speech, kilocalories are alluded to as "calories." All in all, a 2,000-calorie diet really has 2,000 kilocalories of possible energy. One kilocalorie is how much intensity energy expected to raise one kilogram of water from 14.5 to 15.5

°C at one air of strain. One more unit of energy broadly utilized is the joule, which estimates energy with regards to mechanical work. When one kilogram is moved one meter with a force of one newton, the amount of energy required is one joule. The somewhat more elevated levels of energy in human sustenance are bound to be estimated in kilojoules (1 kilojoule = 103 joules) or megajoules (1 megajoule = 106 joules). One kilocalorie is comparable to 4.184 kilojoules.

The energy present in food can be resolved straight by estimating the result of intensity when the food is scorched (oxidized) in a bomb calorimeter. Be that as it may, the human body isn't quite as proficient as a calorimeter, and some potential energy is lost during processing and digestion. Remedied physiological qualities for the warms of ignition of the three energy-yielding supplements, adjusted to entire numbers, are as per the following: 4 kilocalories (17 kilojoules) per gram of carbohydrate; 4 kilocalories (17 kilojoules) per gram of protein; furthermore, fat, 9 kilocalories (38 kilojoules) per gram. Drink liquor (ethyl liquor) additionally yields energy — 7 kilocalories (29 kilojoules) per gram — despite the fact that it isn't fundamental in the eating regimen. Despite the fact that many of them are involved in processes that the body uses to release energy, vitamins, minerals, water, and other components of food have no energy value.

The energy given by a very much processed food can be assessed assuming that the gram measures of energy-yielding substances (non-fiber starch, fat, protein, and liquor) in that food are known. For instance, a cut of white bread containing 12 grams of sugar, 2 grams of protein, and 1 gram of fat supplies 67 kilocalories (280 kilojoules) of energy. Food organization tables and food marks give valuable information to assessing energy and supplement admission of a singular eating routine. Most food varieties give a combination of energy-providing supplements, alongside nutrients, minerals, water, and different substances. Two eminent exemptions are table sugar and vegetable oil, which are basically unadulterated carb (sucrose) and fat, separately.

All through the greater part of the world, protein supplies somewhere in the range of 8 and 16 percent of the energy in the eating regimen, in spite of the fact that there are wide varieties in the extents of fat and sugar in various populaces. In additional prosperous networks around 12 to 15 percent of energy is normally gotten from protein, 30 to 40 percent from fat, and 50 to 60 percent from starch.

Then again, in numerous more unfortunate agrarian social orders, where cereals contain the majority of the eating regimen, carb gives a much bigger level of energy, with protein and fat giving less. The human body is surprisingly versatile and can get by, and even flourish, on generally disparate weight control plans. However, specific health effects are linked to various dietary patterns.

REE and BMR

Energy is required when an individual is truly dynamic as well as in any event, when the body is lying unmoving. Contingent upon a singular's degree of actual work, somewhere in the range of 50 and 80 percent of the energy exhausted every day is dedicated to essential metabolic cycles (basal digestion), which empower the body to remain warm, inhale, siphon blood, and direct various physiological and biosynthetic exercises, remembering blend of new tissue for developing kids and in pregnant and lactating ladies. Absorption and ensuing handling of food by the body likewise utilizes energy and produces heat. This peculiarity, known as the thermic impact of food (or diet-incited thermogenesis), represents around 10% of everyday energy use, shifting fairly with the sythesis of the eating routine and earlier dietary practices. Versatile thermogenesis, one more little yet significant part of energy consumption, reflects modifications in digestion because of changes in surrounding temperature, chemical creation, close to home pressure, or different elements. At long last, the most factor part in energy consumption is actual work, which incorporates practice and other deliberate exercises as well as compulsory exercises, for example, squirming, shuddering, and keeping up with pose. Actual work represents 20 to 40 percent of the all out energy use, even a very dynamic. less in an exceptionally stationary individual and more in somebody.

Basal or resting energy use is associated fundamentally with lean weight (sans fat mass and fundamental fat, barring capacity fat), which is the metabolically dynamic tissue in the body. Very still, organs like the liver, mind, heart, and kidney have the most noteworthy metabolic movement and, consequently, the most significant requirement for energy, while muscle and bone require less energy, and muscle to fat ratio even less. Other than body organization, different elements influencing basal digestion incorporate age, sex, internal heat level, and thyroid chemical levels.

The basal metabolic rate (BMR), an unequivocally characterized proportion of the energy use important to help, not entirely set in stone under controlled and normalized conditions — not long after arousing in that frame of mind, something like 12 hours after the last dinner, and with an agreeable room temperature. Due to pragmatic contemplations, the BMR is seldom estimated; the resting energy consumption still up in the air under less rigid circumstances, with the individual resting serenely around 2 to 4 hours after a feast. By and by, the BMR and REE contrast by something like 10% — the REE is generally somewhat higher — and the terms are utilized conversely.

Energy consumption can be evaluated by direct calorimetry, or estimation of intensity dispersed from the body, which utilizes contraptions, for example, water-cooled pieces of clothing or protected chambers sufficiently enormous to oblige an individual.

Nonetheless, energy use is normally estimated by the less lumbering strategies of circuitous calorimetry, in which intensity delivered by the body is determined from estimations of oxygen breathed in, carbon dioxide breathed out, and urinary nitrogen discharged. The BMR (in kilocalories each day) can be generally assessed utilizing the accompanying recipe: BMR is equal to 70/3 (body mass in kilograms).

The energy expenses of different exercises have been estimated (see table). Strenuous work, on the other hand, may require ten times as many calories per minute as rest. Mental action, however it might appear to be burdening, affects energy prerequisite. A 70-kg (154-pound) man, whose REE throughout a day may be 1,750 kilocalories, could exhaust a sum of 2,400 kilocalories on an exceptionally stationary day and as much as

4,000 kilocalories on an extremely dynamic day. A 55-kg (121-pound) lady, whose day to day resting energy use may be 1,350 kilocalories, could use from 1,850 to in excess of 3,000 complete kilocalories, contingent upon level of action.

This is how the law of energy conservation works: On the off chance that one takes in more energy than is exhausted, over the long run one will put on weight; deficient energy admission brings about weight reduction, as the body taps its energy stores to accommodate prompt requirements. Fat, the body's primary energy reserve in adipose tissue, and glycogen, a short-term storage form of carbohydrate found in muscle and liver, store small amounts of excess food energy. Fat tissue is for the most part fat (around 87%), yet it additionally contains some protein and water. To lose 454 grams (one pound) of fat tissue, an energy shortage of around 3,500 kilocalories (14.6 megajoules) is required.

The human body comprises of materials like those tracked down in food sources; nonetheless, the overall extents vary, as per hereditary directs as well with respect to the one of a kind valuable encounter of the person. A lean man in good health has a body that is roughly 62% water, 16% fat, 16% protein, 6% minerals, and less than 1% carbohydrates. There are also very few vitamins and other random substances in the body. Females for the most part convey more fat (around 22% in a solid lean lady) and somewhat less of different parts than do guys of tantamount weight.

The body's various compartments — lean weight, muscle versus fat, and body water — are continually acclimating to changes in the interior and outside climate with the goal that a condition of dynamic harmony (homeostasis) is kept up with. Tissues in the body are consistently being separated (catabolism) and developed (anabolism) at different rates. For instance, the epithelial cells covering the gastrointestinal system are supplanted at a confounding pace of each and every three or four days, while the life expectancy of red platelets is 120 days, and connective tissue is restored throughout quite a while.

Despite the fact that appraisals of the level of muscle to fat ratio can be made by direct review, this approach is uncertain. Muscle to fat ratio can be estimated by implication utilizing genuinely exact yet exorbitant strategies, for example, submerged gauging, all out body potassium counting, and double energy X-beam absorptiometry (DXA).

Notwithstanding, more reasonable, though less precise, techniques are frequently utilized, for example, anthropometry, in which subcutaneous fat at different locales is estimated utilizing skinfold calipers; bioelectrical impedance, in which protection from a low-force electrical flow is utilized to gauge muscle versus fat; also, close to infrared interactance, in which an infrared light focused on the biceps is utilized to survey fat and protein cooperation. Direct estimation of the body's different compartments must be performed on corpses.

The piece of the body will in general change in fairly unsurprising ways throughout a lifetime — during the developing years, in pregnancy and lactation, and as one ages — with relating changes in supplement needs during various periods of the existence cycle. Standard actual activity can assist with constricting the age-related loss of lean tissue and expansion in muscle to fat ratio.

Carbohydrates, lipids (mostly fats and oils), proteins, vitamins, minerals, and water are the six classes of nutrients found in food. Starches, lipids, and proteins comprise the heft of the eating routine, summing together to around 500 grams (a little more than one pound) each day in genuine weight. These macronutrients supply the raw materials needed to construct and maintain tissues, as well as the fuel needed to carry out the numerous physiological and metabolic processes necessary for life to continue. Conversely, are the micronutrients, which are not themselves energy sources yet work with metabolic cycles all through the body: nutrients, of which people need around 300 milligrams each day in the eating regimen, and minerals, of which around 20 grams each day are required. The last supplement classification is water, which gives the medium in which every one of the body's metabolic cycles happen.

If a nutrient must be obtained from outside the body—typically through food—it is deemed "essential." See table.) These supplements are examined in this part. Despite the fact that they are isolated into classifications for reasons for conversation, one ought to remember that supplements work as a team with one another in the body, not as disconnected substances.

Carbohydrates With 4 kilocalories per gram, carbohydrates—made up of carbon, hydrogen, and oxygen—are the body's primary source of energy. In many sugars, the components hydrogen and oxygen are available in a similar 2:1 proportion as in water, subsequently "carbo" (for carbon) and "hydrate" (for water).

Glucose: The brain, nervous system, and red blood cells primarily use glucose, a simple carbohydrate. Muscle and other body cells can likewise involve glucose for energy, albeit fat is frequently utilized for this reason. Since a consistent stock of glucose is so basic to cells, blood glucose is kept up with inside a generally thin reach through the activity of different chemicals, for the most part insulin, which coordinates the progression of glucose into cells, and glucagon and epinephrine, which recover glucose from capacity.

The body stores a modest quantity of glucose as glycogen, a complex fanned type of starch, in liver and muscle tissue, and this can be separated to glucose and utilized as an energy source during brief periods (a couple of long stretches) of fasting or during seasons of serious active work or stress. On the off chance that blood glucose falls beneath ordinary (hypoglycemia), shortcoming and discombobulation might result. Raised blood glucose (hyperglycemia), as can happen in diabetes, is additionally risky and can't be left untreated.

Glucose can be made in the body from most kinds of starch and from protein, in spite of the fact that protein is normally a costly wellspring of energy. Some negligible measure of sugar is expected in the eating routine — no less than 50 to 100 grams per day. This extras protein as well as guarantees that fats are totally utilized and forestalls a condition known as ketosis, the collection of results of fat breakdown, called ketones, in the body. In spite of the fact that there are extraordinary varieties in the amount and kind of starches eaten all through the world, most weight control plans contain all that could possibly be needed.

Different Sugars and Starch

The least complex carbs are sugars, which give numerous food sources their sweet taste and yet give food to microscopic organisms in the mouth, in this way adding to dental rot. Sugars in the eating routine are monosaccharides, which contain one sugar or saccharide unit, and disaccharides, which contain two saccharide units connected together. Monosaccharides of healthful significance are glucose, fructose, and galactose; Maltose, lactose, and sucrose are all examples of disaccharides. Oligosaccharides, such as raffinose and stachyose, are a slightly more complex type of carbohydrate that has three to ten saccharide units. these mixtures, which are tracked down in beans and different vegetables and can't be processed well by people, represent the gas-creating results of these food sources. Bigger and more intricate stockpiling types of starch are the polysaccharides, which comprise of long chains of glucose units. Starch, the main polysaccharide in the human eating routine — tracked down in grains, vegetables, potatoes, and different vegetables — is comprised of for the most part straight glucose chains (amylose) or predominantly stretching chains (amylopectin). At last, nondigestible polysaccharides known as dietary fiber are found in plant food sources like grains, natural products, vegetables, vegetables, seeds, and nuts.

To be used by the body, all mind boggling starches should be separated into basic sugars, which, thusly, should be separated into monosaccharides — an accomplishment, achieved by catalysts, that beginnings in the mouth and finishes in the small digestive tract, where most retention happens. Each dissacharide is parted into single units by a particular compound; for instance, the chemical lactase separates lactose into its constituent monosaccharides, glucose and galactose. In a large part of the total populace, lactase movement declines during youth and puberty, which prompts a powerlessness to sufficiently process lactose. This acquired characteristic, called lactose narrow mindedness, brings about gastrointestinal distress and loose bowels if an excessive amount of lactose is consumed. The people who have held the capacity to process dairy items proficiently in adulthood are fundamentally of northern European heritage.

Dietary Fiber

Dietary fiber, the primary pieces of plants, can't be processed by the human digestive system in light of the fact that the important catalysts are deficient. With the exception of a small amount that is fermented by bacteria in the large intestine, these compounds that are not digestible pass through the gut unchanged. Despite this, they still contribute to good health. Insoluble fiber doesn't disintegrate in water and gives mass, or roughage, that assists with entrail capability (routineness) and speeds up the exit from the assemblage of possibly cancer-causing or generally hurtful substances in food. Kinds of insoluble fiber are cellulose, most hemicelluloses, and lignin (a phenolic polymer, not a starch). Significant food wellsprings of insoluble fiber are entire grain breads and cereals, wheat grain, and vegetables. The transit time of food through the gut is slowed down by soluble fiber, which dissolves or expands in water. This is an undesirable effect, but it also helps lower blood cholesterol levels (a desirable effect). Gums, pectins, some hemicelluloses, and mucilages are examples of soluble fibers; organic products (particularly citrus leafy foods), oats, grain, and vegetables are significant food sources. Both solvent and insoluble fiber assist with postponing glucose ingestion, subsequently guaranteeing an increasingly slow even inventory of blood glucose. Dietary fiber is remembered to give significant security against a few gastrointestinal infections and to lessen the gamble of other constant illnesses too.

Lipids

Lipids also contain oxygen, hydrogen, and carbon, but they do so in a different way, with significantly fewer oxygen atoms than in carbohydrates. Lipids are dissolvable in natural solvents (like CH3)2CO or ether) and insoluble in water, a property that is promptly seen when an oil-and-vinegar salad dressing isolates rapidly after standing. Triglycerides (fats and oils), phospholipids (like lecithin), and sterols (like cholesterol) are the lipids that are important for nutrition. Lipids in the eating routine vehicle the four fat-solvent nutrients (nutrients A, D, E, and K) and aid their retention in the small digestive system. They likewise convey with them substances that bestow tactile allure and satisfactoriness to food and give satiety esteem, the sensation of being full and fulfilled in the wake of eating a feast. Fats provide an energy yield of 9 kilocalories per gram and are a more concentrated form of energy than carbohydrates. Fat (greasy) tissue in the fat terminals of the body fills in as an energy hold as well as assisting with protecting the body and pad the inner organs.

Fatty Substances

The significant lipids in food and put away in the body as fat are the fatty substances, which comprise of three unsaturated fats joined to a spine of glycerol (a liquor). Unsaturated fats are basically hydrocarbon chains with a carboxylic corrosive gathering (COOH) toward one side, the alpha (α) end, and a methyl bunch (CH3) at the other, omega (ω), end. They are named soaked or unsaturated as indicated by their compound construction. Instead of saturated fatty acids' full complement of hydrogen atoms, a point of unsaturation indicates a double bond between two carbon atoms. A monounsaturated unsaturated fat has one mark of unsaturation, while a polyunsaturated unsaturated fat has at least two.

The table provides a list of the common fatty acids found in foods. The number of carbon atoms in each chain of fatty acids in the human diet and in body tissues can range anywhere from four to 22. Of specific significance for people are the 18-carbon polyunsaturated unsaturated fats alpha-linolenic corrosive (an omega-3 unsaturated fat) and linoleic corrosive (an omega-6 unsaturated fat); these are known as fundamental unsaturated fats since they are expected in limited quantities in the eating regimen. The omega assignments (likewise alluded to as n-3 and n-6) show the area of the main twofold bond from the methyl end of the unsaturated fat. Other unsaturated fats can be orchestrated in the body and are in this way not fundamental in the eating routine. About a tablespoon everyday of a common vegetable oil, for example, safflower or corn oil or a fluctuated diet that incorporates grains, nuts, seeds, and vegetables can satisfy the fundamental unsaturated fat prerequisite. Fundamental unsaturated fats are required for the arrangement of cell films and the amalgamation of chemical like mixtures called eicosanoids (e.g., prostaglandins, thromboxanes, and leukotrienes), which are significant controllers of pulse, blood thickening, and the safe reaction. The utilization of fish a few times per week gives an extra wellspring of omega-3 unsaturated fats that has all the earmarks of being fortifying.

A fat comprising generally of soaked unsaturated fats, particularly lengthy chain unsaturated fats, will in general be strong at room temperature; At room temperature, the fat is liquid if it is mostly composed of unsaturated fatty acids. Fats and oils ordinarily contain combinations of unsaturated fats, albeit the sort of unsaturated fat in most prominent focus normally gives the food its attributes. Margarine and other creature fats are fundamentally soaked; olive and canola oils, monounsaturated; also, fish, corn, safflower, soybean, and sunflower oils, polyunsaturated. In spite of the fact that plant oils will generally be to a great extent unsaturated, there are prominent special cases, for example, coconut fat, which is profoundly immersed yet by the by semiliquid at room temperature in light of the fact that its unsaturated fats are of medium chain length (8 to 14 carbons in length). Above perspective on high protein food sources: chicken, meat, spinach, eggs, nuts, bean, cheddar. (sustenance, wellbeing, food, diet)

Immersed fats will quite often be more steady than unsaturated ones. The food business exploits this property during hydrogenation, in which hydrogen particles are added to a place of unsaturation, consequently making the unsaturated fat more steady and impervious to rancidity (oxidation) as well as more strong and spreadable (as in margarine). Nonetheless, a consequence of the hydrogenation cycle is an adjustment of the state of a few unsaturated fats from a setup referred to as cis to that known as trans. Additionally, trans-fatty acids, which behave more like saturated fatty acids, may have negative effects on health.

Phospholipids

A phospholipid is like a fatty substance with the exception of that it contains a phosphate bunch and a nitrogen-containing compound, for example, choline rather than one of the unsaturated fats. Phospholipids are used as food additives because they are natural emulsifiers, allowing fat and water to mix. In the body, phospholipids permit fats to be suspended in liquids like blood, and they empower lipids to get across cell films starting with one watery compartment then onto the next.

The phospholipid lecithin is ample in food varieties like egg yolks, liver, raw grain, and peanuts. In any case, the liver can combine all the lecithin the body needs in the event that adequate choline is available in the eating regimen.

Sterols

Sterols are extraordinary among lipids in that they have a numerous ring structure. The notable sterol cholesterol is tracked down just in food varieties of creature beginning — meat, egg yolk, fish, poultry, and dairy items. Organ meats (e.g., liver, kidney) and egg yolks have the most cholesterol, while muscle meats and cheeses have less. There are various sterols in shellfish yet not as much cholesterol as was once suspected. Cholesterol is crucial for the construction of cell films and is likewise used to make other significant sterols in the body, among them the sex chemicals, adrenal chemicals, bile acids, and vitamin D. Be that as it may, cholesterol can be orchestrated in the liver, so there is compelling reason need to consume it in the eating routine. Cholesterol-containing stores might develop in the walls of courses, prompting a condition known as atherosclerosis, which adds to myocardial localized necrosis (coronary episode) and stroke. Besides, on the grounds that raised degrees of blood cholesterol, particularly the structure known as low-thickness lipoprotein (LDL) cholesterol, have been related with an expanded gamble of cardiovascular infection, a restricted admission of immersed fat — especially medium-chain soaked unsaturated fats, which act to raise LDL cholesterol levels — is encouraged. Trans-unsaturated fats additionally raise LDL cholesterol, while monounsaturated and polyunsaturated (cis) fats will quite often bring down LDL cholesterol levels. Due to the body's criticism components, dietary cholesterol has just a minor impact on blood cholesterol in a great many people; in any case, since certain people answer unequivocally to cholesterol in the eating routine, a confined admission is frequently encouraged, particularly for those in danger of coronary illness. The perplexing connections between different dietary lipids and blood cholesterol levels, as well as the conceivable wellbeing outcomes of various dietary lipid designs, are talked about in the article wholesome sickness.

Proteins

Proteins, similar to starches and fats, contain carbon, hydrogen, and oxygen, however they likewise contain nitrogen, a part of the amino substance bunch (NH2), and at times sulfur. Proteins act as the fundamental primary material of the body as well as being biochemical impetuses and controllers of qualities. Protein makes up the majority of muscles, bones, internal organs, and the skin, nails, and hair, with the exception of water.

Protein is likewise a significant piece of cell layers and blood (e.g., hemoglobin). Compounds, which catalyze synthetic responses in the body, are additionally protein, as are antibodies, collagen in connective tissue, and a huge number, like insulin.

Tissues all through the body require continuous fix and substitution, and hence the body's protein is turning over continually, being separated and afterward resynthesized on a case by case basis. Together with the proteins in the blood, tissue proteins are in a state of dynamic equilibrium. The diet provides proteins, and the skin, feces, and urine remove proteins. In a sound grown-up, changes are made so how much protein lost is in offset with how much protein ingested. However, the body is in a positive nitrogen balance during times of rapid growth, pregnancy, lactation, recovery from illness, or depletion, as more protein is retained than excreted. The opposite is true during illness or wasting, when more tissue is being broken down than made, leading to a negative nitrogen balance.

Amino Acids

The proteins in food —, for example, egg whites in egg white, casein in dairy items, and gluten in wheat — are separated during absorption into constituent amino acids, which, when assimilated, add to the body's metabolic pool. Amino acids are then joined by means of peptide linkages to collect unambiguous proteins, as coordinated by the hereditary material and because of the body's necessities at that point. Every quality makes at least one proteins, each with a novel grouping of amino acids and exact three-layered setup. Amino acids are additionally expected for the amalgamation of other significant nonprotein compounds, like peptide chemicals, a few synapses, and creatine.

Food contains around 20 normal amino acids, 9 of which are viewed as fundamental, or irreplaceable, for people; i.e., they can't be blended by the body or can't be combined in adequate amounts and subsequently should be taken in the eating regimen. The fundamental amino acids for people are histidine, isoleucine, leucine, lysine, methionine, phenylalanine, threonine, tryptophan, and valine. Restrictively essential amino acids incorporate arginine, cysteine, and tyrosine, which might should be given under extraordinary conditions, like in untimely babies or in individuals with liver illness, due to impeded change from antecedents.

The overall extents of various amino acids differ from one food to another. Good quality, or complete, protein can be found in foods made from animals, such as meat, fish, eggs, and dairy products; i.e., their fundamental amino corrosive examples are like human requirements for protein. (Gelatin, which comes up short on amino corrosive tryptophan, is a special case.) Individual food sources of plant beginning, except for soybeans, are lower quality, or inadequate, protein sources. Lysine, methionine, and tryptophan are the essential restricting amino acids; i.e., they are in littlest stock and in this manner limit how much protein that can be orchestrated. Notwithstanding, a differed veggie lover diet can promptly satisfy human protein prerequisites if the protein-containing food sources are adjusted to such an extent that their fundamental amino acids complete one another. Legumes, like beans, contain a lot of lysine but little methionine, whereas grains have complementary advantages and disadvantages. Consequently, on the off chance that beans and rice are eaten throughout the span of a day, their joint amino corrosive examples will enhance one another and give a more excellent protein than would either food alone. Conventional food designs in local societies have really taken advantage of protein complementarity. Nonetheless, cautious adjusting of plant proteins is important just for those whose protein admission is minor or insufficient. In well-off populaces, where protein admission is significantly in overabundance of necessities, getting adequate great quality protein is normally just a worry for small kids who are not given creature proteins.

Protein Admission

The World Wellbeing Association suggests a day to day admission of 0.75 gram of good quality protein per kilogram of body weight for grown-ups of the two genders. Consequently, a 70-kg (154-pound) man would require 52.5 grams of protein, and a 55-kg (121-pound) lady would require around 41 grams of protein. This proposal, in view of nitrogen balance studies, accepts a satisfactory energy admission. Babies, kids, and pregnant and lactating ladies have extra protein needs to help amalgamation of new tissue or milk creation. Protein prerequisites of perseverance competitors and jocks might be marginally higher than those of inactive people, however this has no down to earth importance since competitors regularly consume substantially more protein than they need.

Protein consumed in overabundance of the body's requirements is corrupted; the nitrogen is discharged as urea, and the leftover keto acids are utilized for energy, giving 4 kilocalories for each gram, or are switched over completely to sugar or fat. During states of fasting, starvation, or deficient dietary admission of protein, lean tissue is separated to supply amino acids for essential body capabilities. Diligent protein deficiency results in sub-standard metabolic capability with expanded chance of contamination and illness.

Nutrients

Nutrients are natural mixtures tracked down in tiny sums in food and expected for typical working — without a doubt, for endurance. People can incorporate specific nutrients somewhat. The skin makes vitamin D, for instance, when it is exposed to sunlight; niacin can be orchestrated from the amino corrosive tryptophan; furthermore, vitamin K and biotin are combined by microscopic organisms living in the stomach. Nonetheless, by and large, people rely upon their eating regimen to supply nutrients. At the point when a nutrient is hard to find or can't be used as expected, a lack of particular disorder results. At the point when the insufficient nutrient is resupplied before irreversible harm happens, the signs and side effects are turned around. The measures of nutrients in food varieties and the sums expected consistently are estimated in milligrams and micrograms.

Not at all like the macronutrients, nutrients don't act as an energy hotspot for the body or give unrefined components to tissue building. Rather, they aid energy-yielding responses and work with metabolic and physiologic cycles all through the body. In addition to its role in vision, vitamin A is necessary for embryonic development, growth, reproduction, proper immune function, and epithelial cell integrity. The B nutrients capability as coenzymes that aid energy digestion; folic corrosive (folate), one of the B nutrients, safeguards against birth surrenders in the beginning phases of pregnancy. L-ascorbic acid assumes a part in building connective tissue as well similar to a cell reinforcement that safeguards against harm by receptive particles (free extremists). Presently viewed as a chemical, vitamin D is engaged with calcium and phosphorus homeostasis and bone digestion. Vitamin E, another cell reinforcement, safeguards against free extreme harm in lipid frameworks, and vitamin K assumes a key part in blood coagulating. Despite the fact that nutrients are frequently examined separately, a significant number of their capabilities are interrelated, and a lack of one can impact the capability of another.

Nutrient classification is fairly complicated, with synthetic names bit by bit supplanting the first letter assignments made in the period of nutrient revelation during the principal half of the twentieth 100 years. Terminology is additionally convoluted by the acknowledgment that nutrients are portions of families with, at times, different dynamic structures. A few nutrients are found in food sources in forerunner frames that should be enacted in the body before they can appropriately satisfy their capability. For instance, beta(β)- carotene, tracked down in plants, is changed over completely to vitamin An in the body.

The 13 nutrients known to be expected by people are arranged into two gatherings as per their solvency. The four fat-dissolvable nutrients (solvent in nonpolar solvents) are nutrients A, D, E, and K. Albeit presently referred to act as a chemical, the enacted type of vitamin D, vitamin D chemical (calcitriol), is as yet gathered with the nutrients too. The nine water-dissolvable nutrients (dissolvable in polar solvents) are L-ascorbic acid and the eight B-complex nutrients: thiamin, riboflavin, niacin, vitamin B6, folic corrosive, vitamin B12, pantothenic corrosive, and biotin. Choline is a nutrient like dietary part that is plainly expected for ordinary digestion however that can be combined by the body. Although it has not been established that choline is essential to the diet of humans throughout their lives, it may be necessary in the diet of premature infants and possibly those with certain medical conditions.

Different vitamins are more or less susceptible to being destroyed by chemicals and the environment. For instance, thiamin is particularly defenseless against drawn out warming, riboflavin to bright or glaring light, and L-ascorbic acid to oxidation (as when a piece of natural product is cut open and the nutrient is presented to air). When compared to fat-soluble vitamins, water-soluble vitamins generally break down more quickly when cooked.

A vitamin's solubility has an impact not only on where it is found in foods but also on how the body absorbs, transports, stores, and excretes it. Except for vitamin B12, which is provided by just food sources of creature beginning, the water-dissolvable nutrients are blended by plants and tracked down in both plant and creature food varieties. Severe veggie lovers (vegetarians), who eat no food varieties of creature beginning, are along these lines in danger of lack of vitamin B12. Fat-solvent nutrients, then again, are tracked down in relationship with fats and oils in food varieties and in the body and commonly require protein transporters for transport through the water-filled compartments of the body.

Water-dissolvable nutrients are not obviously put away in that frame of mind (with the exception of vitamin B12) and in this way should be drunk routinely in the eating regimen. On the off chance that taken in overabundance they are promptly discharged in the pee, despite the fact that there is potential poisonousness even with water-dissolvable nutrients; particularly critical in such manner is vitamin B6. Since fat-dissolvable nutrients are put away in the liver and greasy tissue, they don't be guaranteed to must be taken in day to day, inasmuch as normal admissions over the long run — weeks, months, or even years — address the body's issues. Nonetheless, the way that these nutrients can be put away expands the chance of poisonousness assuming exceptionally enormous dosages are taken. This is especially of worry with nutrients An and D, which can be poisonous whenever taken in overabundance. There are accepted medical uses for pharmacological (or "megadose") levels of some vitamins, which are many times higher than the amount typically found in food. Niacin, for instance, is utilized to bring down blood cholesterol levels; Psoriasis can be treated with vitamin D; what's more, pharmacological subsidiaries of vitamin An are utilized to treat skin inflammation and other skin conditions as well as to reduce skin wrinkling. Nonetheless, utilization of nutrients or other dietary enhancements in sums fundamentally in abundance of suggested levels isn't exhorted without clinical oversight.

Nutrients blended in the research center are similar atoms as those extricated from food, and they can't be recognized by the body. However, not all forms of a vitamin are created equal. Vitamin E supplements with the label "natural" or "d-tocopherol" typically contain more vitamin E activity than those with the label "dl-tocopherol." Vitamins that are found in food have a distinct advantage over vitamins that are found in supplements because they are associated with other substances that might be beneficial and have a lower risk of toxicity. Supplements for nutrition cannot replace a healthy diet.

Minerals

In contrast to the complicated natural mixtures (carbs, lipids, proteins, nutrients) examined in past segments, minerals are basic inorganic components — frequently as salts in the body — that are not themselves processed, nor are they a wellspring of energy. About half of the body's minerals are calcium and one quarter are phosphorus (phosphates), with the other essential minerals, which must come from food, making up the remaining 4% to 6%. Minerals bestow hardness to bones and teeth as well as capability extensively in digestion — e.g., as electrolytes controlling the development of water all through cells, as parts of catalyst frameworks, and as constituents of numerous natural atoms.

As supplements, minerals are customarily isolated into two gatherings as per the sums present in and required by the body. The significant minerals (macrominerals) — those expected in measures of 100 milligrams or more each day — are calcium, phosphorus (phosphates), magnesium, sulfur, sodium, chloride, and potassium. The minor components (microminerals or minor elements), expected in a lot more modest measures of around 15 milligrams each day or less, incorporate iron, zinc, copper, manganese, iodine (iodide), selenium, fluoride, molybdenum, chromium, and cobalt (as a feature of the vitamin B12 particle). Although a strictly essential function in human nutrition has not been established, fluoride is considered a beneficial nutrient for its role in preventing dental caries.

The term ultratrace components is once in a while used to portray minerals that are tracked down in the eating routine in tiny amounts (micrograms every day) and are available in human tissue too; these incorporate arsenic, boron, nickel, silicon, and vanadium. The precise function of these and other ultratrace elements (such as tin, lithium, and aluminum) in human tissues and their significance for human health are unknown, despite their roles being demonstrated in experimental animals.

Minerals have assorted capabilities, including muscle compression, nerve transmission, blood thickening, insusceptibility, the upkeep of circulatory strain, and development and advancement. The significant minerals, except for sulfur, ordinarily happen in the body in Ionlc (charged) structure: sodium, potassium, magnesium, and calcium as certain particles (cations) and chloride and phosphates as bad particles (anions). Mineral salts broke up in body liquids assist with directing liquid equilibrium, osmotic strain, and corrosive base equilibrium.

In ionic forms like sulfate, sulfur also has important functions, but most of the sulfur in the body is nonionic and is an essential component of certain organic molecules like the B vitamins thiamin, biotin, and pantothenic acid and the amino acids methionine, cysteine, and cystine. Other mineral components that are constituents of natural mixtures incorporate iron, which is essential for hemoglobin (the oxygen-conveying protein in red platelets), and iodine, a part of thyroid chemicals, which assist with controlling body digestion. Phosphate groups can also be found in a lot of organic molecules, like the high-energy molecule adenosine triphosphate (ATP), genetic material (DNA and RNA), and phospholipids in cell membranes.

The degrees of various minerals in food varieties are affected by developing circumstances (e.g., soil and water piece) as well as by how the food is handled. Minerals are not annihilated during food planning; as a matter of fact, a food can be singed totally and the minerals (debris) will stay unaltered. In any case, minerals can be lost by draining into cooking water that is hence disposed of.

Mineral absorption and, as a result, body availability are influenced by numerous factors. By and large, minerals are preferred assimilated from creature food varieties over from plant food varieties. The latter include fiber and additional substances that hinder absorption. Cereal grains and legumes are the main sources of phytic acid, which can make some minerals insoluble and thus indigestible by forming complexes with them. Just a little level of the calcium in spinach is consumed in light of the fact that spinach likewise contains a lot of oxalic corrosive, which ties calcium. A few minerals, especially those of a comparable size and charge, contend with one another for retention. For instance, iron supplementation might decrease zinc retention, while unnecessary admissions of zinc can slow down copper assimilation. Then again, the assimilation of iron from plants (nonheme iron) is upgraded when L-ascorbic acid is all the while present in the eating regimen, and calcium retention is further developed by sufficient measures of vitamin D. Another key component that impacts mineral retention is the physiological requirement for the mineral at that point.

Not at all like numerous nutrients, which have a more extensive security range, minerals can be poisonous on the off chance that taken in portions not far above suggested levels. This is especially true for the trace elements like copper and iron. Unplanned ingestion of iron enhancements has been a significant reason for lethal harming in small kids.

Water

Albeit frequently disregarded as a supplement, water (H2O) is really the most basic supplement of all. People can endure a long time without food yet just only days without water.

Water gives the medium in which supplements and side-effects are moved all through the body and the bunch biochemical responses of digestion happen. Water takes into account temperature guideline, the upkeep of circulatory strain and blood volume, the design of enormous atoms, and the unbending nature of body tissues. Additionally, it serves as a solvent, a lubricant (in joints), and a cushion of protection (in the eye, spinal fluid, and amniotic fluid). The progression of water all through cells is exactly constrained by moving electrolyte fixations on one or the other side of the cell film. Potassium, magnesium, phosphate, and sulfate are basically intracellular electrolytes; Extracellular sodium and chloride are major ones.

Water makes up around 50 to 70 percent of body weight, roughly 60% in solid grown-ups and a considerably higher rate in kids. Since lean tissue is around 3/4 water, and greasy tissue is something like one-fifth water, body organization — how much fat specifically — decides the level of body water. Men typically have more lean tissue than women do, so a greater proportion of their weight is water.

Not only is water consumed as water and in other beverages, but it is also a major component of many foods, particularly fruits and vegetables, which may contain 85 to 95% water. Water additionally is made in the body as a final result of digestion. Around 2.5 liters (around 2.6 quarts) of water are turned over day to day, with water discharge (basically in pee, water fume from lungs, sweat misfortune from skin, and excrement) adjusting admission from all sources. Since water necessities differ with environment, level of movement, dietary arrangement, and different elements, there is nobody suggestion for day to day water consumption. Adults, on the other hand, typically require at least 2 liters (8 cups) of water per day from all sources. Thirst isn't dependable as a register for parchedness, which commonly happens before the body is provoked to supplant liquid. As a result, it's a good idea to drink water throughout the day, especially in hot weather, when you sweat more, when you exercise a lot, when you're sick, or when you're in a dehydrating situation like flying.

Nutrition Types

The accompanying nine nutrition types reflect food varieties with by and large comparable healthful qualities:

1. Cereals,
2. Dull roots,
3. Vegetables,
4. Vegetables and organic products,
5. Sugars, jam, and syrups,
6. Meat, fish, and eggs,
7. Endlessly milk items,
8. Fats and oils, and
9. Refreshments.

Grains

The oats are grasses that have been reproduced over centuries to bear enormous seeds (i.e., grain). The main cereals for human utilization are rice, wheat, and corn (maize). Others incorporate grain, oats, and millet. The starch rich cereals contrast well and the protein-rich food varieties in energy esteem; moreover, the expense of creation (per calorie) of oats is not exactly that of practically any remaining food sources and they can be put away dry for a long time. Hence, the vast majority of the world's weight control plans are organized to meet fundamental calorie prerequisites from the less expensive starch food sources. Starch makes up the majority of all grains. Oats have a remarkable 9% fat content, making them one of the lowest-fat cereals. How much protein in grains goes from 6 to 16 percent yet doesn't have as high a nutritive worth as that of numerous creature food sources in view of the low lysine content.

Discussion exists with regards to the general benefits of white endlessly bread produced using entire wheat flour. White flour contains only a small amount of the germ (embryo) and the outer coverings (bran), but it contains approximately 72% of the grain. Since the B nutrients are packed for the most part in the scutellum (covering of the microorganism), and less significantly in the wheat, the vitamin B content of white flour, except if falsely advanced, is not exactly that of earthy colored flour. Dietary fiber is found for the most part in the grain, so that white flour contains around 33% of that in entire wheat flour. White flour is mandatorily improved with engineered nutrients in various nations, including the US and the Unified Realm, so the nutrient substance is like that of the hazier flours. White flour, obviously, still needs fiber and any yet unidentified advantageous elements that might be available in the external layers of the wheat.

B nutrients are likewise lost when earthy colored rice is cleaned to yield white rice. Individuals living on white rice and little else are in danger of fostering the illness beriberi, which is brought about by a lack of thiamin (vitamin B1). Beriberi used to be common in poor Asian communities where polished rice made up a lot of the food. With the increased availability of other foods and, in some regions, the addition of thiamin to rice, the disease has virtually disappeared from Asia.

Yellow corn varies from different oats in that it contains carotenoids with vitamin A movement. (Carotene, the precursor to vitamin A, can be found in genetically modified so-called golden rice.) Corn also contains less tryptophan than other cereals. The niacin in corn is in a bound structure that can't be processed or consumed by people except if pretreated with lime (calcium hydroxide) or except if youthful grains are eaten at the supposed smooth stage (for the most part as sweet corn). Niacin is also produced in the body as a metabolite of the amino acid tryptophan; however, when the tryptophan content is too low, this alternative source is unavailable.

Starchy roots Potatoes, sweet potatoes, yams, taro, and cassava are examples of starchy roots that are commonly consumed in large quantities. Their nutritive worth overall looks like that of oats. The potato, notwithstanding, gives some protein (2%) and furthermore contains L-ascorbic acid. The yellow-fleshed assortments of yam contain the shade beta-carotene, convertible in the body into vitamin A. Cassava is very low in protein, and most assortments contain cyanide-shaping mixtures that make them harmful except if handled accurately.

Vegetables

Beans and peas are the seeds of leguminous harvests that can use barometrical nitrogen by means of parasitic microorganisms appended to their underlying foundations. Vegetables contain no less than 20% protein, and they are a decent wellspring of the greater part of the B nutrients and of iron. Like cereals, most vegetables are low in fat; a significant special case is the soybean (17%), a significant business wellspring of palatable oil. Tofu, or bean curd, is produced using soybeans and is a significant wellspring of protein in China,

Japan, Korea, and Southeast Asia. Peanuts (groundnuts) are likewise the seeds of a leguminous plant, in spite of the fact that they mature underground; a large part of the yield is handled for its oil.

Vegetables and Organic Products

Vegetables and organic products have comparative nutritive properties. Since 70% or a greater amount of their weight is water, they give relatively little energy or protein, however many contain L-ascorbic acid and carotene. Notwithstanding, cooked vegetables are a dubious wellspring of L-ascorbic acid, as this nutrient is effectively obliterated by heat. The dim green verdant vegetables are especially great wellsprings of vitamin A movement. Vegetables likewise give calcium and iron yet frequently in a structure that is ineffectively consumed. The more average natural products, like apples, oranges, and berries, are wealthy in sugar. Bananas are a decent wellspring of potassium. Vegetables and organic products additionally contain fiber, which adds mass to the gastrointestinal substance and is valuable in forestalling blockage.

Organically, nuts are really a sort of natural product, yet they are very divergent in character with their hard shell and high fat substance. When dried, the coconut, for instance, has about 60% fat. Another fat-rich fruit, olives are typically grown for their oil.

Sugars, Jam, and Syrups

One quality of diets of prosperous social orders is their high happy of sugar. This is expected to some extent to sugar added at the table or as a fixing in treats, saves, and improved colas or different refreshments. Foods also contain sugars that are naturally occurring (lactose in milk and fructose, glucose, and sucrose in some fruits and vegetables). Sugar, in any case, contains no protein, minerals, or nutrients and hence has been known as the wellspring of "void calories."

Sugar is an excellent preservative because it adsorbs water and prevents the growth of microorganisms. Fruit can be preserved by making jam or marmalade, but the majority of the vitamin C is lost, and the products can be up to 70% sugar. Honey and regular syrups (e.g., maple syrup) are made out of in excess of 75% sugar.

Meat, Fish, and Eggs

For the most part meats comprise of around 20% protein, 20% fat, and 60 percent water. How much fat present in a specific part of meat differs extraordinarily, with the sort of meat as well as with the quality; the "energy esteem" shifts in direct extent with the fat substance . Meat is significant for its protein, which is of high organic worth. Pork is a phenomenal wellspring of thiamin. Meat is likewise a decent wellspring of niacin, vitamin B12, vitamin B6, and the mineral supplements iron, zinc, phosphorus, potassium, and magnesium. Liver is the capacity organ for, and is extremely plentiful in, vitamin A, riboflavin, and folic corrosive. In many societies the organs (offal) of creatures — including the kidneys, the heart, the tongue, and the liver — are viewed as delights. Liver is an especially rich wellspring of numerous nutrients.

The strong tissue of fishes comprises of 13 to 20 percent protein, fat going from under 1 to in excess of 20%, and 60 to 82 percent water that changes conversely with fat substance (see table). Numerous types of fish, for example, cod and haddock, move fat in the liver and thus have very lean muscles. The tissues of other fish, like salmon and herring, may contain 15% fat or more. However, in contrast to the fat found in animal products, fish oil contains a lot of essential long-chain fatty acids, especially eicosapentaenoic acid.

Endlessly Milk Items

The milk of every types of creature is a finished nourishment for its young. In addition, one pint of cow's milk contains approximately

90% of the calcium, 30%-40% of the riboflavin, 25%-30% of the protein, 10%-20% of the calories, vitamins A and B, and up to 10% of the iron and vitamin D an adult needs.

Human bosom milk is the ideal nourishment for babies, gave it comes from a sound, very much fed mother and the newborn child is full-term. Bosom milk contains significant antibodies, white platelets, and supplements. In people group where cleanliness is poor, bosom took care of children have less diseases than equation took care of infants. Infants who were unable to breastfeed were previously given cow's milk that had been partially "humanized" by adding water and a small amount of sugar or wheat flour. Nonetheless, this was a long way from an ideal substitute for bosom milk, being lower in iron and containing undenatured proteins that could deliver unfavorably susceptible responses with seeping into the stomach and, at times, dermatitis.

Lactose, the trademark sugar of milk, is a disaccharide made of the monosaccharides glucose and galactose. A few grown-ups can separate the lactose of enormous amounts of milk into galactose and glucose, however others have an acquired lactose narrow mindedness because of the lactase catalyst done being discharged into the stomach after the time of weaning. Therefore, unabsorbed lactose is aged by microorganisms and produces swelling and gas. Individuals who have little lactase in their bodies can in any case polish off a lot of milk in the event that it has been permitted to turn sour, in the event that lactobacilli have parted the vast majority of the lactose into lactic corrosive (as in yogurt), or on the other hand on the off chance that the lactose has been treated with monetarily accessible lactase. Individuals beginning in northern Europe normally hold full digestive lactase movement into grown-up life.

Most economically accessible milk has been sanitized with intensity to kill cow-like tuberculosis creatures and other potential microbes. The most generally involved technique for purifying milk is the high-temperature, brief time frame (HTST) sanitization treatment. On the off chance that items are to be put away under refrigeration, or even at room temperature, for significant stretches of time, they might be handled by ultrahigh temperature (UHT) sanitization. One more strategy for safeguarding milk without refrigeration includes the evacuation of water to frame dense milk, which can be presented to air for a few days without decay. Milk, either entire or defatted, can likewise be dried to a powder. In certain nations, for example, the US, milk is homogenized so that fat particles are separated and equitably conveyed all through the item.

Cow's milk is great nourishment for human grown-ups, yet the cream (i.e., the fat) contains 52% immersed unsaturated fats as contrasted and just 3% polyunsaturated fat. This fat is either plastered with the milk or eaten in spread or cream. Since milk fat is viewed as unfortunate by individuals who need to decrease their energy admission or cholesterol level, the dairy business has grown low-fat cow's milk (with 2% fat rather than the just about 4% of entire milk), exceptionally low-fat skim milk, and skim milk with extra nonfat milk solids (lactose, protein, and calcium) that give more body to the milk. Buttermilk, initially the watery buildup of margarine making, is currently produced using either low-fat or skim milk that has been vaccinated with nonpathogenic microbes.

Cheddar making is an old craftsmanship previously utilized on ranches to change over excess milk into a food that could be put away without refrigeration. Rennet is an enzyme that is found in the stomach of a calf. When it is added to milk, it causes the milk protein casein to coagulate into a semisolid substance known as curd, which holds most of the fat. The leftover watery fluid (whey) is then depleted, and the curd is salted, immunized with nonpathogenic creatures, and permitted to dry and develop. Cheddar is wealthy in protein and calcium and is a decent wellspring of vitamin An and riboflavin. Most cheeses, in any case, contain around 25 to 30 percent fat (comprising around 70% of the calories of the cheddar), which is for the most part immersed, and they are normally high in sodium.

Butter, suet (beef fat), lard (pork fat), and fish oils are the animal fats that humans use. Learn the difference between saturated and polyunsaturated fats Learn the difference between saturated and polyunsaturated fatsSee all videos for this article Significant vegetable oils incorporate olive oil, nut (groundnut) oil, coconut oil, cottonseed oil, sunflower seed oil, soybean oil, safflower oil, assault oil, sesame (gingelly) oil, mustard oil, red palm oil, and corn oil. Fats and oils give a bigger number of calories per gram than some other food, yet they contain no protein and barely any micronutrients. Just margarine and the recently referenced fish-liver oils contain any vitamin An or D, however red palm oil contains carotene, which is switched over completely to vitamin An in the body. Nutrients

An and D are added to margarines. Every normal fat and oils contain variable measures of vitamin E, the fat-dissolvable nutrient cancer prevention agent.

The prevalent substances in fats and oils are fatty substances, synthetic mixtures containing any three unsaturated fats joined with a particle of glycerol. A fatty acid is considered saturated when it lacks double bonds; with the presence of at least one twofold securities, an unsaturated fat is supposed to be unsaturated. Fats with a high level of immersed unsaturated fats, e.g., margarine and fat, will generally be strong at room temperature. Those with a high level of unsaturated fats are typically fluid oils, e.g., sunflower, safflower, and corn oils. The course of hydrogenation is utilized by the food business to switch unsaturated oils over completely to immersed strong fats, which are more impervious to rancidity. Be that as it may, hydrogenation additionally causes the arrangement of trans-unsaturated fats. These seem to have a portion of similar bothersome consequences for blood cholesterol as soaked unsaturated fats.

The diet needs a small group of fatty acids. They happen in body structures, particularly the various layers inside and around cells, and can't be combined in that frame of mind from different fats. Linoleic corrosive is the most significant of these unsaturated fats since it is convertible to other fundamental unsaturated fats. Linoleic acid is a polyunsaturated fatty acid with two double bonds. As well just like a fundamental unsaturated fat, it will in general lower the cholesterol level in the blood. Linoleic corrosive happens in moderate to high extents in a large number of the seed oils, e.g., corn, sunflower, cottonseed, and safflower oils. A few margarines (polyunsaturated margarines) utilize a mix of oils chose to give a modestly high linoleic corrosive substance.

Beverages Although the majority of adults consume between one and two liters (roughly one and two quarts) of water each day, the majority of this intake comes from beverages like coffee, tea, fruit juices, and soft drinks. As a general rule, these are valued something else for their taste or for their belongings than for their nutritive worth. Natural product juices are valuable for their L-ascorbic acid substance and are great wellsprings of potassium; notwithstanding, they will quite often be exceptionally high in sugar. Tea and coffee have little nutritional value on their own; espresso contains some niacin, and tea contains fluoride and manganese. These refreshments likewise contain normal caffeine, which makes an invigorating difference. Coca-Colas contain caffeine, and so-called diet soft drinks substitute artificial sweeteners for sugars in small amounts to reduce their calorie content.

Since ethyl liquor (ethanol) has an energy worth of 7 kilocalories for every gram, extremely huge measures of energy can be acquired from cocktails (see table). Wines have 10 to 13% alcohol, beer has 2% to 6%, and most spirits have up to 40%. Champagne and dessert wines may have sugar added to them, and fermented drinks also contain a lot of sugar that remains. With a couple of special cases, cocktails contain no supplements and are just a wellspring of "void calories." The main nutrient present in huge sums in brew is riboflavin. Wines are absent any trace of nutrients yet here and there contain a lot of iron, likely obtained from iron vessels utilized in their planning. Malnutrition is known to be more likely in people who drink a lot of alcohol because it can damage the gut's ability to absorb nutrients and because heavy drinkers often skip meals. Then again, proof from various examinations shows that people polishing off one to two beverages each day are more grounded than are the individuals who swear off drinking liquor. This may be expected to a limited extent to substances in red wine, for example, flavonoids and tannins, which might safeguard against coronary illness.

Recommendations for Dietary and Nutrient Intake

The notions of what constitutes a healthy diet change with time, geography, custom, and an evolving understanding of nutrition.

Previously, individuals needed to live for the most part on food that was privately created. With industrialization and globalization, be that as it may, food can now be moved over significant distances. Scientists should be cautious in making speculations about a public eating regimen from a moderately little example of the populace; the poor can't bear to eat a similar eating routine as the rich, and numerous nations have huge outsider gatherings with their own particular food designs. Indeed, even inside a culture, certain individuals go without on moral or strict grounds from eating specific food varieties. People who live in more prosperous nations typically consume more meat and other animal products. By examination, the eating regimens of those living in more unfortunate, agrarian nations depend fundamentally on cereals as wheat flour, white rice, or corn, with creature items giving under 10% of energy.

One more distinction between societies is the degree to which dairy items are consumed. Dairy products, for instance, account for about 2% of the energy consumed by the Chinese. Dairy products, on the other hand, account for nearly 10% of Pakistan's energy. Among Western weight control plans, the most minimal in immersed fat is the supposed Mediterranean eating routine. During the 1950s it was found that Europeans living in rustic regions close to the Mediterranean Ocean had a more noteworthy daily routine hope than those experiencing somewhere else in Europe, notwithstanding unfortunate clinical benefits and a lower expectation for everyday life. The customary eating regimen of Mediterranean people groups is low in creature items; all things being equal, olive oil is a significant wellspring of monounsaturated fat. Likewise, tomatoes and green verdant vegetables, which are consistently consumed in huge amounts in the district, contain an assortment of cell reinforcement intensifies that are believed to be fortifying.

Since the publication of dietary goals for the Nordic countries in 1968 and the United States in 1977, a number of nations have established dietary goals and guidelines. These goals and guidelines have been revised on a regular basis as a means of translating scientific recommendations into dietary suggestions that are easy to follow and can be implemented immediately. These definitive assertions — a few distributed by logical bodies and some by government organizations — expect to advance long haul wellbeing and to forestall or lessen the possibilities creating persistent and degenerative illnesses. The most recent dietary recommendations include variations on the following fundamental themes, despite the fact that the guidelines of various nations may differ in significant ways: eat different food varieties; perform normal actual work and keep a sound weight; limit utilization of immersed fat, trans fat, sugar, salt (all the more explicitly, sodium), and liquor; furthermore, accentuate vegetables, organic products, and entire grains.

Food Guide Pyramids and Different Guides

Various organizations for dietary objectives and rules have been created throughout the years as instructive devices, gathering food varieties of comparable supplement content together to assist with working with the choice of a reasonable eating routine. In the US, the four nutritional category plan of the 1950s —

which recommended a milk bunch, a meat bunch, a products of the soil bunch, and a breads and grains bunch as a fundamental eating routine — was supplanted in 1992 by the five significant nutrition types of the Food Guide Pyramid. This visual showcase, which has its underlying foundations in an aide created in Sweden during the 1970s, was presented by the US Branch of Horticulture (USDA) as a device for assisting people in general with developing an everyday example of savvy food decisions, going from liberal utilization of grain items, as addressed in the wide base of the pyramid, to saving utilization of fats, oils, and sweet food sources, as addressed in the zenith. The Asian, Latin American, Mediterranean, and even vegetarian diets—all of which place an emphasis on grains, vegetables, and fruits— all saw the development of similar appliances. While a transformation of the 1992 USDA pyramid was utilized by Mexico, Chile, the Philippines, and Panama, a rainbow was utilized by Canada, a square by Zimbabwe, plates by Australia and the Unified Realm, a bean pot by Guatemala, the number 6 by Japan, and a pagoda by South Korea and China.

USDA MyPyramid dietary guidelines Numerous nations altered the visual representation of their food guides at the beginning of the 21st century. For instance, in 2005 Japan presented a turning top food guide that basically was an upset variant of the U.S. pyramid realistic. The USDA also published new dietary guidelines in the same year. The original Food Guide Pyramid, which was called MyPyramid and featured vibrant vertical stripes of varying widths to represent the proportions of various food groups, was also redesigned. The MyPyramid graphic used a figure climbing steps, much like Japan's spinning-top graphic, which showed a figure running on the top's upper level. This was done to show how important it is to exercise every day. Not at all like the first Food Guide Pyramid, the theoretical calculation of MyPyramid didn't offer explicit dietary direction initially; rather, people were coordinated to an intelligent Site for tweaked eating plans in view of their age, sex, and movement level.

In 2011 the USDA deserted MyPyramid and presented MyPlate, what partitioned the four essential nutrition classes (organic products, grains, protein, and vegetables) into segments on a plate, with the size of each segment addressing the general dietary extents of every nutritional category. A little circle displayed at the edge of the plate was utilized to delineate the dietary consideration and extent of dairy items. Not at all like MyPyramid, MyPlate did exclude an activity part, nor did it incorporate a segment for fats and oils. The two were comparative, in any case, in that the direction they offered was vague and was upheld by a Site.

Adjusting Rules to Culture

Dietary rules have been generally the territory of additional prosperous nations, where amending awkward nature because of overconsumption and improper food decisions has been vital. Not until 1989 were proposition for dietary rules distributed according to the viewpoint of low-pay nations, like India, where the essential sustenance issues originated from the absence of chance to obtain or eat required food. However, even in such nations, a small but growing number of wealthy individuals who had adopted some of the dietary practices of the industrialized world were at an increased risk of obesity and chronic disease. For instance, the Chinese Dietary Rules, distributed by the Chinese Nourishment Society in 1997, made suggestions for that piece of the populace managing healthful sicknesses like those subsequent from iodine and lacks of vitamin A, for individuals in a few far off regions where there was an absence of food, as well concerning the metropolitan populace adapting to evolving way of life, dietary overabundance, and expanding paces of constant illness. The traditional Chinese diet of cereals served as the foundation for the Food Guide Pagoda, a visual representation meant to assist Chinese consumers in following the dietary recommendations. The individuals who couldn't endure new milk were urged to polish off yogurt or other dairy items as a wellspring of calcium. The Chinese did not consume a lot of sugar, so the pagoda did not include it, unlike Western diet recommendations; nonetheless, kids and teenagers specifically were advised to restrict sugar consumption in view of the gamble of dental caries.

sUPPLEMENT SUGGESTIONS

The generally basic dietary rules examined above give direction to dinner arranging. Norms for assessing the sufficiency of explicit supplements in a singular eating regimen or the eating routine of a populace require more point by point and quantitative proposals. Supplement suggestions not entirely settled by logical bodies inside a country at the command of government organizations. The World Wellbeing Association and different organizations of the Assembled Countries have likewise given provides details regarding supplements and food parts. The U.S. National Academy of Sciences first published the Recommended Dietary Allowances (RDAs) in 1941, and they were updated every few years until 1989. These dietary guidelines were used to evaluate populations' nutritional intakes and plan food supplies. In establishing amounts of various nutrients sufficient to meet the nutritional requirements of the majority of healthy individuals, the RDAs reflected the best scientific judgment of the time.

Dietary Reference Admissions

During the 1990s a change in outlook occurred as researchers from the US and Canada united in an aggressive long term task to rethink dietary principles for the two nations. In the overhauled approach, known as the Dietary Reference Admissions (DRIs), exemplary signs of lack, like scurvy and beriberi, were viewed as a deficient reason for suggestions. Where justified by an adequate exploration base, the rules depend on pointers with more extensive importance, those that could mirror a diminished gamble of persistent sicknesses like osteoporosis, coronary illness, hypertension, or disease. DRIs are meant to help people plan a healthy diet and avoid eating too much of a particular nutrient. The DRIs' all-encompassing strategy has been a model for other nations. A DRI report was distributed in 1997, and resulting refreshes were distributed for explicit supplements and for some food parts, for example, flavonoids that are not viewed as supplements but rather affect wellbeing.

Human Respiratory Framework

Human respiratory framework, the framework in people that takes up oxygen and removes carbon dioxide.

The Structure of the Respiratory System

The human gas-exchanging organ, the lung, is in the thorax, where the bony and muscular thoracic cage protects its delicate tissues. The lung gives the tissues of the human body with a nonstop progression of oxygen and gets the blood free from the vaporous side-effect, carbon dioxide. Environmental air is siphoned in and out consistently through an arrangement of lines, called leading aviation routes, which get the gas-trade district together with the beyond the body. There are two types of airway systems: upper and lower.

The progress between the two frameworks is found where the pathways of the respiratory and stomach related frameworks cross, right at the highest point of the larynx.

The upper aviation route framework includes the nose and the paranasal depressions (or sinuses), the pharynx (or throat), and somewhat likewise the oral pit, since it could utilized for relax. The lower aviation route framework comprises of the larynx, the windpipe, the stem bronchi, and every one of the aviation routes ramifying seriously inside the lungs, like the intrapulmonary bronchi, the bronchioles, and the alveolar conduits. It is obvious that other organ systems need to work together for respiration. The stomach, as the super respiratory muscle, and the intercostal muscles of the chest wall assume a fundamental part by creating, heavily influenced by the focal sensory system, the siphoning activity on the lung. The muscles grow and get the inside space of the chest, the hard system of which is shaped by the ribs and the thoracic vertebrae. The mechanics of breathing explains how the ribs and muscles of the chest wall and lung contribute to respiration. The blood, as a transporter for the gases, and the circulatory framework (i.e., the heart and the veins) are required components of a functioning respiratory framework.

Morphology of the Upper Aviation Routes

The nose

The nose is the outside bulge of an interior space, the nasal cavity. It is partitioned into a left and right channel by a slight average cartilaginous and hard wall, the nasal septum. Each channel opens to the face by a nostril and into the pharynx by the choana. The floor of the nasal depression is shaped by the sense of taste, which likewise frames the top of the oral pit. The mind boggling state of the nasal pit is because of projections of hard edges, the predominant, center, and mediocre turbinate bones (or conchae), from the parallel wall. The ways consequently shaped underneath each edge are known as the unrivaled, center, and second rate nasal meatuses.

Attributes of the Human Body

On each side, the intranasal space speaks with a progression of adjoining air-filled holes inside the skull (the paranasal sinuses) and furthermore, by means of the nasolacrimal pipe, with the lacrimal contraption toward the edge of the eye. The lacrimal fluid enters the nasal cavity through the duct. This reality makes sense of why nasal breath can be quickly disabled or even blocked during sobbing: In addition to overflowing into tears, the lacrimal fluid is also flooding the nasal cavity.

The paranasal sinuses are sets of matched single or various pits of variable size. The majority of their improvement happens after birth, and they arrive at their last size toward age 20. The sinuses are situated in four different skull bones — the maxilla, the front facing, the ethmoid, and the sphenoid bones. Correspondingly, they are known as the maxillary sinus, which is the biggest pit; the sinus in the front the ethmoid sinuses; and the sphenoid sinus, which is in the nasal cavity's upper, posterior wall. The sinuses have two chief capabilities: since they are loaded up with air, they assist with keeping the heaviness of the skull inside sensible cutoff points, and they act as reverberation chambers for the human voice.

The nasal hole with its contiguous spaces is lined by a respiratory mucosa. Regularly, the mucosa of the nose contains bodily fluid emitting organs and venous plexuses; its top cell layer, the epithelium, comprises basically of two cell types, ciliated and discharging cells. The particular ancillary functions of the nose and the upper airways as a whole in relation to respiration are reflected in this structural design. They clean, soak, and warm the motivated air, setting it up for cozy contact with the fragile tissues of the gas-trade region. The process of drying and cooling the air during nasal exhalation conserves energy and water.

The lining of the nasal cavity is different in two places. The vestibule, at the entry of the nose, is lined by skin that bears short thick hairs called vibrissae. The sensory epithelium of the olfactory bulb checks the quality of the inspired air in the roof of the nose. From the olfactory cells, approximately two dozen olfactory nerves transmit the sense of smell to the central nervous system via the bony roof of the nasal cavity.

The Pharynx

For the physical portrayal, the pharynx can be partitioned into three stories. The upper floor, the nasopharynx, is basically a way for air and discharges from the nose to the oral pharynx. Through auditory tubes that open on both sides, it also connects to the middle ear's tympanic cavity. The demonstration of gulping opens momentarily the typically imploded hear-able cylinders and permits the center ears to be circulated air through and pressure contrasts to be balanced. The pharyngeal tonsil is a lymphatic organ that is located in the nasopharynx's posterior wall. At the point when it is amplified (as in tonsil hypertrophy or adenoid vegetation), it might impede nasal breath and adjust the reverberation example of the voice.

The center floor of the pharynx associates anteriorly to the mouth and is consequently called the oral pharynx or oropharynx. It is delimited from the nasopharynx by the delicate sense of taste, which rooftops the back piece of the oral depression.

The lower floor of the pharynx is known as the hypopharynx. Its front wall is framed by the back piece of the tongue. Lying straight over the larynx, it addresses the site where the pathways of air and food cross one another: Air from the nasal hole streams into the larynx, and food from the oral depression is steered to the throat straightforwardly behind the larynx. The epiglottis, a cartilaginous, leaf-molded fold, capabilities as a top to the larynx and, during the demonstration of gulping, controls the traffic of air and food.

The larynx

The larynx is an organ of perplexing construction that serves a double capability: as an air waterway to the lungs and a regulator of its entrance, and as the organ of phonation. Sound is created by driving air through a sagittal cut shaped by the vocal ropes, the glottis. The air column above the vocal cords as well as the vocal cords themselves vibrate as a result of this. As confirmed via prepared vocalists, this capability can be firmly controlled and finely tuned. Control is accomplished by various muscles innervated by the laryngeal nerves. For the exact capability of the solid contraption, the muscles should be secured to a settling structure. The laryngeal skeleton comprises of just about twelve bits of ligament, the majority of them tiny, interconnected by tendons and layers. The biggest ligament of the larynx, the thyroid ligament, is made of two plates melded anteriorly in the midline. At the upper finish of the combination line is a cut, the thyroid score; The laryngeal prominence is a forward projection below it. Both of these designs are effectively felt through the skin. The point between the two ligament plates is more honed and the conspicuousness more set apart in men than in ladies, which has provided this design with the normal name of Thyroid cartilage.

Behind the shieldlike thyroid ligament, the vocal strings range the laryngeal lumen. They are similar to elastic ligaments that are attached anteriorly in the angle of the thyroid shield and posteriorly to the arytenoid cartilages, which are two small, pyramidal pieces of cartilage. The vocal ligaments are a part of an elastic tissue tube that looks like an organ pipe. Simply over the vocal strings, the epiglottis is likewise appended to the rear of the thyroid plate by its tail. The cricoid, one more enormous cartilaginous piece of the laryngeal skeleton, has a seal ring shape. The larynx's posterior wall houses the ring's broad plate and the anterior wall houses the narrow arch. The cricoid is situated beneath the thyroid ligament, to which it is participated in an enunciation supported by tendons. The cross over hub of the joint permits a hingelike turn between the two ligaments. This movement changes the distance between the cricoid plate and the shield of the thyroid cartilage by tilting it. Since the arytenoid ligaments lay upstanding on the cricoid plate, they follow its shifting development. This system assumes a significant part in changing length and strain of the vocal ropes. By articulating with the cricoid plate, the arytenoid cartilages are able to rotate and slide to open and close the glottis.

Seen visually, the lumen of the laryngeal cylinder has an hourglass shape, with its tightest width at the glottis. Simply over the vocal strings there is an extra sets of mucosal folds called the misleading vocal ropes or the vestibular folds. Like the genuine vocal strings, they are likewise framed by the free finish of a fibroelastic layer. Between the vestibular folds and the vocal strings, the laryngeal space augments and structures sidelong pockets stretching out vertical. This space is known as the ventricle of the larynx.

Since the hole between the vestibular folds is dependably bigger than the hole between the vocal lines, the last option can undoubtedly be seen from above with the laryngoscope, an instrument intended for visual review of the inside of the larynx.

The strong device of the larynx includes two practically particular gatherings. The natural muscles act straightforwardly or in a roundabout way on the shape, length, and strain of the vocal ropes. The extraneous muscles follow up on the larynx in general, moving it vertical (e.g., during sharp phonation or gulping) or descending. The inborn muscles connect to the skeletal parts of the actual larynx; The laryngeal skeleton is connected to the hyoid bone or the pharynx cranially and caudally to the sternum (breastbone) by extrinsic muscles.

The Windpipe and the Stem Bronchi

Beneath the larynx lies the windpipe, a cylinder around 10 to 12 cm (3.9 to 4.7 inches) long and 2 cm (0.8 inch) wide. Its wall is hardened by 16 to 20 trademark horseshoe-formed, fragmented ligament rings that open rearward and are implanted in a thick connective tissue. A thick layer of transverse smooth muscle fibers stretches across the cartilage gap in the dorsal wall. The inside of the windpipe is lined by the regular respiratory epithelium. The mucosal layer contains mucous organs.

At its lower end, the windpipe partitions in an altered Y into the two stem (or primary) bronchi, one each for the left and right lung. The right primary bronchus has a bigger measurement, is situated all the more in an upward direction, and is more limited than the left principal bronchus. The commonsense result of this plan is that unfamiliar bodies passing past the larynx will ordinarily slip into the right lung. The stem bronchi have a similar structure to the trachea.

Underlying Model of the Aviation Route Tree

The order of the partitioning aviation routes, and part of the way likewise of the veins infiltrating the lung, to a great extent decides the interior lung structure. Practically the intrapulmonary aviation route framework can be partitioned into three zones, a proximal, simply leading zone, a fringe, simply gas-trading zone, and a temporary in the middle between, where the two capabilities grade into each other. According to a morphological perspective, be that as it may, it's a good idea to recognize the somewhat thick-walled, simply air-directing cylinders from those parts of the aviation route tree basically intended to allow gas trade.

Because the branching pattern affects air flow and particle deposition, the structural design of the airway tree is important for its function. It is generally agreed that the rules of irregular dichotomy apply when modeling the human airway tree. Standard polarity implies that each part of a treelike construction leads to two girl parts of indistinguishable aspects. In unpredictable polarity, nonetheless, the little girl branches might contrast extraordinarily long and measurement. The models compute the typical way from the windpipe to the lung outskirts as comprising of around 24-25 ages of branches. Individual ways, in any case, may go from 11 to 30 ages. If the trachea is counted as generation 0, the transition between the respiratory and conductive portions of an airway occurs, on average, at the end of the 16th generation. The trachea, the two stem bronchi, the bronchi, and the bronchioles are the conducting airways. Their capability is to additionally warm, soak, and clean the motivated air and convey it to the gas-trading zone of the lung. They are fixed by the commonplace respiratory epithelium with ciliated cells and various sprinkled bodily fluid emitting challis cells. Ciliated cells are available far down in the aviation route tree, their level diminishing with the restricting of the cylinders, as does the recurrence of cup cells. In bronchioles the cup cells are totally supplanted by one more sort of secretory cells named Clara cells.

Printed in the USA
CPSIA information can be obtained
at www.ICGtesting.com
LVHW011734060824
787515LV00008B/460